MANAGEMENT OF PATIENTS WITH CHRONIC PAIN

MANAGEMENT OF PATIENTS WITH CHRONIC PAIN

Edited by

STEVEN F. BRENA, M.D.
Department of Rehabilitation Medicine and Anesthesiology
Director, Pain Control Center
Emory University
Atlanta, Georgia

STANLEY L. CHAPMAN, Ph.D.
Department of Rehabilitation Medicine
Emory University
Atlanta, Georgia

MTP PRESS LIMITED
International Medical Publishers

Published in the UK and Europe by
MTP Press Limited
Falcon House
Lancaster, England

Published in the US by
SPECTRUM PUBLICATIONS, INC.
175-20 Wexford Terrace
Jamaica, NY 11432

Softcover reprint of the hardcover 1st edition 1983

ISBN-13: 978-94-011-6313-2 e-ISBN-13: 978-94-011-6311-8
DOI: 10.1007/978-94-011-6311-8

Preface

This book has been written for the general health care professional, from every medical and paramedical specialization. Because pain is the most common factor driving patients to seek professional advice, it is likely that every physician, psychologist, and therapist has been clinically exposed to the difficulty and the frequent frustration of dealing with people in pain. All of them may find in this book some explanations for their puzzles and some updated information, which usually are published in specialized journals not ordinarily read by the general practitioner.

Actually the book has been addressed to professionals at two different levels of general practice. At one level is the busy practitioner who treats most patients with "acute" pain, and who may use this information in daily practice to prevent the onset of chronic pain; a common effort from all professionals currently is needed to curb the "epidemic" of chronic pain in the United States. At another level the book has been addressed to the practitioner who may have a more intense desire to become involved in the actual management of chronic pain patients.

The book is roughly divided into three sections: the first six chapters deal with definitions and concepts of pain, and with basic information about the neurophysiology and the psychology of pain. Chapters 7 and 8 describe in some detail certain pain syndromes most commonly seen in general practicce. In these two chapters, the material has not been ordered according to *traditional etiologies,* but rather according to *pain mechanisms;* this approach affords a clearer understanding of the physiological factors underlying clinical phenomena. The second section (Chapters 9, 10, and 11) describes the diagnostic process in pain problems; again the material is not presented according to traditional etiological diagnosis, but rather it describes a comprehensive pathological, psychological, and operational process for the evaluation and the classification of chronic pain states. The third section (Chapters 12–21) critically reviews treatment modalities presently available for management of chronic pain. Chapter 22 has been added to provide health practitioners with a brief insight into the process of law for pain-disabled patients, which often becomes intertwined with general practice and affects the behaviors and the health of patients involved.

Many data are presented to support the points that have been made; the bulk of evidence from the literature has been "filtered"—so to speak—to extract the pertinent facts and some classical ''pearls'' of medical information, without overloading the text with excessive references. Considerable information also is provided through the clinical and research findings from the Emory University Pain Control Center.

The core of the message contained in this book in some ways may be shocking to the general practitioner; many cases of chronic pain represent a veritable ''sensory'' disability, not dissimilar in neurophysiological and psychological mechanisms from the motor disability of patients with central injuries impairing the musculoskeletal system.

The editors wish to thank the contributors for their efforts in pouring out into their respective chapters a knowledge distilled from their clinical and academic experience. A circular, comprehensive vision of the complexity of pain could not have been achieved without their valuable cooperation.

Grateful thanks are also addressed to the secretaries of the Emory Pain Control Center, Edna Davis and Leigh Tinker, who spent so much overtime in typing and retyping the manuscript; without their faithful cooperation, it would have been hard to meet the challenge of writing a book.

Finally, a warm thanks should go to the members of our own families, for their loving patience and understanding during the long evenings and weekend hours spent in the solitude of the office, reading, writing, and editing.

Steven F. Brena
Stanley L. Chapman
Atlanta, 1982

Table of Contents

List of Contributors

KENNETH V. ANDERSON, Ph.D.
Professor of Anatomy
Chairman, Department of Anatomy
University of Mississippi
Jackson, Mississippi

BONNIE M. BLOSSOM, R.P.T.
Chief Physical Therapist
Center for Rehabilitation Medicine
Emory University
Atlanta, Georgia

STEVEN F. BRENA, M.D.
Professor of Rehabilitation Medicine
and Anesthesiology
Director, Pain Control Center
Emory University
Atlanta, Georgia

RENE CAILLIET, M.D.
Professor and Chairman
Rehabilitative Medicine Department
University of Southern California
School of Medicine
Los Angeles, California

STANLEY L. CHAPMAN, Ph.D.
Senior Associate, Psychology
Department of Rehabilitation
Medicine
Emory University
Atlanta, Georgia

BENJAMIN L. CRUE, M.D.
Clinical Professor of Neurological
Surgery
University of Southern California
Los Angeles, California
Director, New Hope Pain Center
Alhambra, California

BETTE A. GROAT, M.A., O.T.R.
Chief Occupational Therapist
Emory University Hospital
Emory University
Atlanta, Georgia

HOWARD I. GROSSMAN, A.B.,
L.L.B., L.L.M.
Administrative Law Judge
Decatur, Georgia

WILLIAM D. HAMMONDS, M.D.
Assistant Professor of
Anesthesiology
and Rehabilitation Medicine
Emory University
Atlanta, Georgia

STEPHEN J. JOHNSON, Ph.D.
Instructor, Psychology
Department of Rehabilitation
Medicine
Emory University
Atlanta, Georgia

RICHARD H. MORSE, M.D.,
M.P.H.
Director, Mercy Hospital Center for
Chronic Pain and Disability
Rehabilitation
Louisiana State University Medical
School
New Orleans, Louisiana

VADDADI RAO, M.D.
Assistant Professor of Rehabilitation
Medicine
Chief of Division, Grady Memorial
Hospital
Emory University
Atlanta, Georgia

JAMES ROUTON, M.D.
Director, Atlanta Pain Control Center
Crawford Long Hospital
Emory University
Atlanta, Georgia

STEVEN L. WOLF, Ph.D., R.P.T.
Associate Professor of Rehabilitation
Medicine
Emory University
Atlanta, Georgia

1

The Mystery of Pain: Is Pain a Sensation?

STEVEN F. BRENA

Pain is the most puzzling problem in general practice. Semantic and existential definitions of pain and a brief critical review of current medical points of view are presented. A "black box" model to understand pain in terms of observable sets of phenomena is discussed. Inputs into the "black box"–the human central nervous system–are both biological and environmental, unconditioned and learned. Five factors commonly identified in chronic pain patients are discussed–the so-called "five-D's syndrome of learned pain." Pathogenic pain and learned pain are defined as interrelated phenomena along a linear spectrum of nociceptive events.

Pain is one of the most puzzling problems in the practice of medicine. In its acute form it seems to be clearly related to many well-recognized disease processes, but in its chronic form it often defies medical knowledge and most current treatment modalities. Paradoxically those same therapies, such as drugs and surgical interventions, which seem to relieve the painful experience associated with well-defined biological disorders, quite often result in physical and emotional deterioration in chronic sufferers.

The problem of pain is not confined behind the closed doors of clinics and hospitals; quite often it spills over and invades the offices of other professionals, such as claims adjusters, vocational counselors, and attorneys. Eventually it finds its way into the courtrooms of the law.

Chronic pain, however, is not a modern-age phenomenon. One of the best descriptions of a chronic sufferer can be found in the *New Testament*: " . . . a certain woman, which had an issue of blood twelve years, and had suffered many things of many physicians and had spent all she had, and was nothing bettered, but rather grew worse" (King James version—Mark 5:25–26).

The word "pain" is derived from a Sanskrit root, *Pu*, meaning sacrifice, and from the Latin word, *poena*, meaning punishment. In its semantic origin, the experience of pain clearly implies the concept of retribution of religious significance in which human suffering is veiwed as a process of penance and atonement for trespass against natural or Divine laws. The ancient Greeks, and the Romans after them, had no concept of pain as a neurological phenomenon; although they were aware of the brain and of the spinal cord, they were not aware of the central nervous system as a functional unit. They viewed the experience of pain as a phenomenon involving the totality of our being, or as a "passion of the soul" as Aristotle called it. They were not alone in this way of thinking; the Hindus, the ancient Egyptians, and the Jews have left several written testimonies bearing witness to the belief that pain is mainly an emotional and existential experience. For example, in the Lamentations of Jeremiah we can read a vivid description of what we would call a "psychosomatic conversion" of an emotional distress into physical symptoms. Jeremiah is lamenting upon the fate of Israel gone into political havoc, " . . . mine eyes do fail with tears, my bowels are troubled, my liver is poured upon the earth" (King James version—Lamentations of Jeremiah, 2:11).

During the 15 centuries between the fall of Rome and the modern age, Greek thought greatly influenced the development of Christian thinking. The concept of pain as a passion of the soul was accepted and human suffering was accounted for as punishment for sins against religious rules and dogmas. Even during the Renaissance, despite improved knowledge of the anatomy of the brain, spinal cord, and peripheral nervous system, little effort was made to give an anatomical and physiological basis to the painful experience. René Descartes, despite his attempt to fit the function of the human body into his mechanistic philosophy, denied the existence of sensory nerves for perception of pain. Characteristically he viewed pain as an expression of an excessive state of awareness appreciated only in the soul "within the pineal gland" (Keele, 1957).

Not until the 19th century, soon after Johannes Müeller wrote about his theory of specific nerve energy (Bonica, 1953) did scientists focus their attention on the experimental analysis of pain. Soon the pendulum swung to the other direction. At the beginning of the 20th century, a great bulk of work was produced to support the idea that pain was nothing but a physical sensation, a kind of sixth sense, not much different from the other five human senses, with its own specific neurological, cable-like apparatus designed to provide information about tissue damages. The new ideas carried with them a new optimism that dominated most of the first half of this century's thinking: If pain is indeed a sensation, it should be controlled by acting upon its pathological courses and blocking its nervous pathways. The sensory cable-like model proved to be useful in treating pain associated with surgery and acute illness, but it failed in each attempt for long-term control of the painful experience associated with chronic sickness, and even less to relieve the suffering from emotional distress.

A review of the current medical literature reveals a great deal of confusion and frustration concerning issues involving pain. From one side, the biomedical model, which views pain as the consequence of biological bodily changes, is quite successful in controlling numerous pathological processes, eventually restoring biological function to normality. On the other side, the removal of known pathological processes is not always followed by restoration to health in the whole individual, nor does the return to normal physical functions necessarily relieve the painful experience.

At the same time, research and studies on pain have begun to show how elusive and complex this phenomenon is. If, indeed, there is a neurological apparatus subserving the perception of pain, its activity appears to be subject to a large number of variables—both excitory and inhibitory, emotional and biological—which may profoundly affect the painful experience itself, quite independently of any organic disease entity.

Moreover, over the centuries we have worked ourselves into many semantic traps and puzzles that cloud and often cripple our objective dealings with chronic sufferers. An example of such traps would be the question "Is pain real?" and the concept of "organic pain versus psychogenic pain." Short of clear-cut evidence of malingering, every painful experience must be assumed to be "real" to the individual sufferer, in the presence of, as well as in the absence of, organic pathology; as in all sensory perceptions, pain involves an interplay between physical sensations and their emotional and cognitive interpretations. Each individual is prone to view the painful experience and to interreact with other individuals who complain of pain, according to his/her own personality, feelings, and philosophy of life. We cannot escape these existential interreactions; health professionals must be carefully aware of their own emotions and attitudes to minimize the clouding of their judgments.

The issue of the "reality" of pain, as well as of all our sensory perceptions, has challenged the thinking of philosophers throughout the ages and yet has not been solved. Probably Leibnitz was quite right when he stated that each individual is a "monad," a completely closed unit, whose existence is separate from outer experiences. In other words, Leibnitz seemed to view our sensory perceptions as being totally inadequate to generate knowlege of the outer physical world. After him, Kant elaborated upon the same concept, when he wrote that "the real thing"—i.e., the true nature of the physical world (the *Noumenon*)— cannot be known through sensory investigation. Our senses can only grasp the "phenomenical" aspect of things as they appear to our sensory perceptions. Modern relativistic physics dramatically corroborated the philosophy of Kant, when it was discovered that the so-called "subatomic particles" are processes rather than objects, whose pattern of activity is affected by the very fact that an investigator has set up an experiment to observe them (Capra, 1977).

As physicians we must be aware of a similar phenomenon when we interact with a patient: The process of interaction itself effects changes that are quite

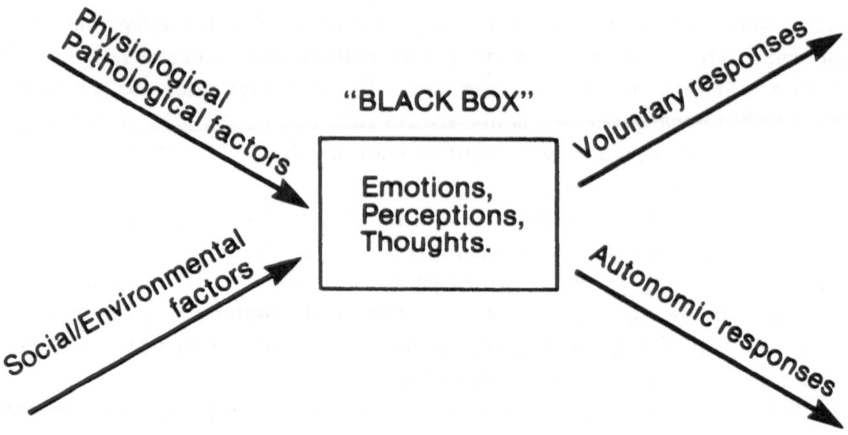

FIG.1-1. The black box model

independent of any treatment modality; such a process is involved in the so-called "placebo effect." A negative patient–doctor interaction may also trigger a "nocebo" effect (Latin *nocere*, to damage, to hurt), where a patient seems to deteriorate despite all successful therapeutic efforts to treat the biomedical disorder.

Probably the most effective way to avoid semantic traps and intellectual puzzles is to look at the phenomenon of pain with the eyes of a scientist in cybernetics and consider the so-called "black box model." The "black box" represents the sufferer who is experiencing "something" within. Unless there is some kind of communication, no one else can know what the sufferer is experiencing: But as soon as the patient starts to communicate, that patient will also start to interact with others; and the interaction itself will interfere with the effectiveness of the communication as a faithful descriptor of the intimate black box experience. For example, the pain complaint of the patient in the doctor's office, where the expectation is "relief" and "cure," may be quite different from the behavior of the same patient in a courtroom, where the expectation is economic reward for the verbalized "painful" discomfort.

In the black box model, an observer can only make statements about inputs to the black box, outputs from the box, and the relationship between the two sets of data (Fig. 1-1).

Inputs to black boxes—human beings in all their complexity—are not only of a physiological and pathological nature (nociceptive and unconditioned),[1] but

[1]*Editors' note*: For the sake of classification, physiological and pathological stimuli may be considered *unconditioned*; however, it must be understood that physiological phenomena can also be *conditioned* through a process of learning, as research on biofeedback has amply demonstrated

are also determined by a history of learning from the family, culture, and society (environmental and conditioned). Examples of environmental stimuli may include inactivity, excused release from anxiety-producing pressures, weather conditions, the desire for drugs, and any other of an infinite number of socioeconomic cues. Pathological nociception is triggered by changes in tissue homeostasis. Several causative mechanisms may be responsible: (1) metabolic derangements, leading to the accumulation of abnormal metabolites that act as irritants; (2) circulatory abnormalities, including changes in arterial blood flow leading to conditions of regional ischemia, and changes in venous return, leading to increased intravascular pressure, which squeezes fluid out of the vascular bed, producing swelling and edema; (3) visceral malfunction of any bodily organ, leading to organic derangements pertinent to the biological role of the disease organ; (4) mechanical compression, infiltration, and destruction of nervous and other deep somatic structures, compression and/or occlusion of blood vessels, and compression and/or occlusion of a viscus; and (5) exogenous mechanical, thermal, and chemical stimulation of such intensity as to cause injury.

Output factors include a large number of responses mediated through voluntary and the autonomic neuromuscular systems, vocal (which is a voluntary muscular behavior) and nonvocal.

Conditioned factors are always interplaying in any given situation, providing a continuous learning experience from infancy to old age, which profoundly affects any subsequent events. How well this existential experience is integrated is a nonmeasurable function of the black box itself.

To consider the pain complaints of a patient recently injured at work or in an automobile accident as simple and true indicators of tissue damage is quite an oversimplification, since in that particular emergency the person is likely to pour in all past experiences learned in other related events. However, in that time-limited situation of acute and emergency medicine, most of the conditioned factors can be safely disregarded so that efforts may be effectively concentrated to correct the nociceptive pathological damage; in such situations some changes in the related output variables can be rightly expected. This statement is true, but not completely true, since even in acute medicine, nocebo and placebo effects play important roles in effecting changes. Moreover a large number of biological functions whose changes medicine takes as indicators of physiological derangements are also under the continuous influence of ecological factors, such as circadian and other space–time rhythms (NIMH, 1970).

In chronic illness and chronic pain states, the impact of conditioned factors is enormous, quite often outweighing the role of nociceptive stimulation. Through learning, pain complaints, the obsessive search for "pain-relieving" drugs, postural and gait abnormalities, inactivity and unemployment can persist in excess of, or in the absence of, demonstrable pathological lesions.

Brena and Chapman (1981) have proposed the term "learned pain syndrome'' to emphasize that learned pain is indeed a disease entity with deep existential roots, which profoundly upsets the physical, emotional, and social balance of the chronic sufferer.

Learned pain can be detected in chronic sufferers by the presence of five well-defined groups of symptoms (the so-called ''five D's'').

THE FIVE D'S

Dramatization of Complaints

The average patient is usually capable of describing a painful experience in clear crisp terms (''I have a deep, dull ache right here.'') On the other hand, patients with learned pain are likely to describe their discomfort in a diffuse and generalized manner and to choose words with high emotional impact (''I hurt all over,'' ''My back is on fire,'' or ''My head is ready to burst open,'' etc.) Dramatic shifts of complaints often are seen at different times, and in different places or situations. For example, a patient with learned pain may report to one physician a dramatic ''pain relief,'' only to notify another physician or an attorney a few days later that he/she ''was hurting like being in Hell.'' Dramatic pain complaints and desperate pleas for help in cases of learned pain may lead to unnecessary medical interventions with no results other than further to establish patients in their sick roles.[2]

Dysfunction

Various musculoskeletal impairments can be caused by misuse of braces, collars, and ambulatory devices, leading to multiple postural and gait abnormalities. The unnecessary use of such devices can also be a kind of ''badge'' to wear in order to be well recognized as a sick or disabled person. Poor postural habits and low levels of daily activity may lead to contractures and myofibrositis in disused muscles (Chapter 7); prolonged periods of inactivity can cause osteoporosis, overweight, and circulatory and respiratory disorders. Vasomotor and sudomotor disturbances, altered motility, and secretion of the gastrointestinal tract may be the consequence of hyperactivity of the neurovegetative system from various emotional maladjustments.

Many patients with learned pain report decreased sexual drive and performance (Chapter 13); various sexual dysfunctions can also be related to

[2]Unpublished data presented to the first World Congress of the International Association for Studies of Pain (1975); ''Social and Environmental Factors in the Experience of Pain'' by O'Donnell, Brena, and Crawford

misuse of depressant medications. Through changes in homeostasis, many dysfunctional syndromes become at the same time a source of added nociceptive stimulation. In addition inactivity is associated with increased psychological depression and further identification with the sick role.

Drug Misuse

The single most common and devastating problem for chronic sufferers is misuse of various drugs usually prescribed for acute, pathogenic pain and anxiety. Cross-reactions and side effects from general and peripheral analgesics, sedatives, and antianxiety agents severely tax the biological and psychological balance of the individual sufferer, often resulting in added nociceptive damage, such as aspirin-related gastritis and phenacetin-related kidney damage (Chapter 12).

Dependency

People in pain show a tendency to give up self-reliance and let themselves be controlled by the environment. Through the slow process of "learned helplessness" (Chapter 6), they have lost the capability to cope and to control their lives. Many of them float miserably from doctors' to attorneys' offices with no real understanding of the needs for and results of such visits.

Disability

The definition of disability implies not only degrees of body impairment, but also issues of age, education, motivation, and culture. Within the context of chronic pain, disability can be defined as dependency upon a source of income that is contingent upon continuing pain complaints and claims to be sick. Disability benefits, pending litigation, and the desire for early disability as retirement pension are strong pain reinforcers.[3] In a sample population of 141 patients at the Emory Pain Control Center, 33 percent were Workers Compensation clients and 18 percent were patients with pending litigation for automobile and other accidents.[4]

Paid disability plays an important role in conditioning patients' responses to treatment. It may actually deter injured workers from returning to normal activities and gainful employment (Chapters 10 and 14).

[3] "Liberal Payments Prolong Disabilities," *Health Insurance News*, August 29, 1979

[4] Unpublished data

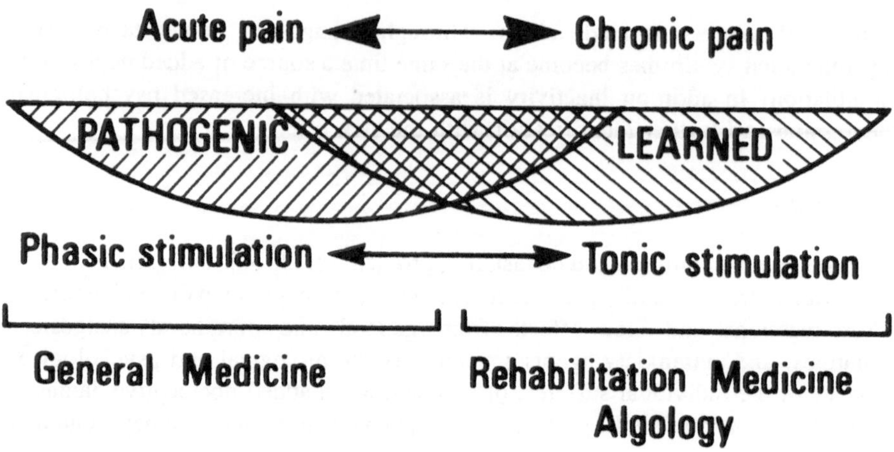

FIG. 1-2. The nociceptive spectrum. Modified from Brena, S.F., Chapman, S.L. 1982. Chronic pain: an algorithm for management. Postgrad. Med. 72:111–117.

CONCLUSIONS

In conclusion the phenomenon of pain may be viewed as a linear spectrum of nociceptive events, ranging from pathogenic pain to learned pain with a large overlapping area between the two opposite sides (Fig. 1-2).

Pathogenic pain may be defined as a painful perception, primarily sustained by a well-identified biomedical abnormality, which triggers "phasic" and episodic, nociceptive stimulation of varying degrees of intensity, frequency, and duration. At the other end of the spectrum, learned pain may be defined as a painful experience from predominant socioemotional factors, either in the presence of a "tonic" steady nociception from a nonprogressive, noninvasive, pathological focus, or in the absence of any identifiable nociceptive stimulation.*

The black box model provides an adequate operational definition of the chronic pain patient in terms of observable phenomena. Short of further research findings in the biochemistry of pain, it also provides the best available approach for classification and measurement of chronic pain states. Reference to this model will be made throughout the course of this book, when issues relating to the diagnosis of chronic pain patients are discussed.

**Editors' note*: The terms "pathogenic pain" and "learned pain" have some similarity with the currently accepted definition of "organic pain" and "psychogenic pain." They have the distinct advantage of pinpointing the primary mechanism of the pain syndrome, that is, pathological nociception versus learning

REFERENCES

Bonica, J.J. 1953. *The Management of Pain*. Philadelphia: Lea & Febiger, p. 23.

Brena, S.F., and Chapman, S.L. 1981. The learned pain syndrome. *Postgrad. Med.* 69: 53–64.

Capra, F. 1977. *The Tao of Physics*. New York: Quality Book Club.

Keele, K.D. 1957. *Anatomies of Pain*. Oxford: Blackwell.

National Institute of Mental Health. 1970. *Biological Rhythms in Psychiatry and Medicine*. Washington, D.C.: U.S. Department of Health, Education and Welfare.

2

Pain Control Facilities: Roots, Organization, and Function

STEVEN F. BRENA

Chronic pain results in an intolerable wastage of human and economic resources. The roots of this enormous problem are briefly discussed. Highlights in the evolution of the concept that chronic pain is a disease state of its own are mentioned. Health and illness behaviors are defined and presented as variables independent from biomedical findings. Pain-control facilities are defined; their structure, organization, and function outlined; and supportive data presented.

THE COST OF PAIN

Figures quoted by John Bonica (1979) indicate that the cost of chronic pain is staggering, in terms both of human suffering and of economic loss. About 75 million Americans suffer from some kind of chronic pain. Backaches alone afflict 23 million and another 24 million suffer severe headaches. Their disabilities result in the loss of approximately 700 million workdays every year. The total cost of chronic pain in terms of lost production, medication, hospitalization, and professional fees totals about $57 billion per year.

A study of 80 subjects by Brena et al. (1981) at the Emory University Pain Control Center seems to indicate that the overall cost of chronic pain is even greater than the figures presented by Bonica. The study was composed of a sample of 55 men and 25 women (mean age = 39.9) drawn from the patient population at the Emory Center. The data are presented in Table 2-1.

These figures would suggest that the loss of wages combined with social support systems could cost the taxpayer from $15,000 to $24,000 per individual per year.

One million pain-disabled patients per year would then cost an average of $20 billion per year. How many Americans per year are pain-disabled is hard to estimate, considering the multitude of agencies that administer disability funds: private institutions for injured workers, the Social Security Fund, the Veterans

Table 2-1
(A) Unit of Economic Loss for Pain-Disabled Subjects

Average Income Loss		Average Tax Loss	
Per week:	$ 207	Per week:	$ 41
Per year:	$9,936	Per year:	$1,968

(B) Unit of Costs for Disability Income and Medical Expenses for Pain-Disabled Subjects

Income Support Benefits	Yearly	Medical Costs (Average)	Yearly
Georgia Workmen's Compensation	$ 5,720	Hospital per diem	$ 1,918
SSDI Benefits — family of four	$14,100	Surgical expenses:	
		Laminectomy (range $5,000–$10,000)	$ 7,500

Administration, etc. The Social Security Administration alone estimates that the total number of beneficiaries for 1980 is five million Americans, up from two million in 1971 with a rate of growth ten times faster than the growth of the general population. (Grossman, 1980). If only 2 percent of the total U.S. population were disabled by pain every year, the economic cost to the taxpayer, without medical expenses, would be in excess of $80 billion. A further analysis of the 80 selected subjects at Emory found that 60 percent of them would be able to return to gainful employment compatible with their age, education, previous work history, and work skills, if they were properly managed, medically and vocationally.

THE PROBLEM IN PERSPECTIVE

The roots of this enormous socioeconomic problem are deeply embedded in the philosophy of present-day health care in the Western culture, which still accepts the Cartesian model of dualism between mind and body. This school of thought maintained the total separation of the body from the mind (which Descartes confused with the soul), permitting an intensive study of the body and leading to enormous advances in science and medicine by enabling the scientist to focus research on *matter* (of which the body is a mechanical part) without bothering about the working of the *mind*. As a result a biomedical disease model was developed, which considers any disease process as an episodic consequence of an accidental mechanical breakdown.

The biomedical model has developed into a well-tuned system for understanding and treating the disease process, using molecular biology as its basic scientific discipline. The success in treating acute diseases has profoundly changed the mortality and morbidity situation around the world. Many acute diseases have been almost wiped out, to the point that chronic diseases, many of them related to the process of aging, are now predominant. In chronic illness, however, the biomedical model seems to work much less efficiently. There is an increasing awareness that critical factors contributing to the morbidity of chronic illness are as much related to social and behavioral factors as they are to the degree of tissue pathology. Yet Western traditional medicine usually relegates emotional and environmental factors to a minimal role, if any.

The World Health Organization has broadened the definition of health to include not merely the absence of disease, but also "a state of complete physical, emotional and social well-being." These concepts can be extrapolated to form certain definitions: (1) *health behavior*—normal activities of daily living (ADL), no drug dependence, self-reliance, and the ability to carry on normal social roles; and (2) *illness behavior*—low ADL, excessive reliance on drugs, dependence, and inability to carry on normal social roles. Social modeling can promote illness behavior in excess of, or even in the absence of, biomedical findings through a process of conditioning and vicarious learning. Conversely health behavior can exist in the presence of disease as the example of millions of fully functioning individuals with various degrees of tissue damage demonstrates every day. Emphasis on the disease process as the only cause of illness behavior has led millions of individuals to consider themselves disabled and drug dependent in a socially acceptable way, promoting excessive and costly searches for elusive pathological findings to justify the continuing illness behavior.

The phenomenon of pain is a typical example to illustrate this point. Pain is an existential experience universally associated with the natural process of living, aging, and dying. Biomedicine has transformed it into a symptom of disease; to explain it contemporary science has evolved from the cablelike neurological conceptualization of the earlier decades of this century toward the search for a "molecular analog for pain" (as Ng has called it), which will "wipe out" every "pain" by providing new classes of more potent drugs or devices (Ng, 1980).

The biomedical conceptualization of pain is per force reflected in present legislation regulating the granting of disability benefits: if pain is a symptom of disease, the pain-disabled patient should be granted a temporary disability status and then allowed to wait in paid idleness, perhaps for years, until the disease has been identified and eliminated. The adversary legal system in the United States is ideal for keeping a worker who has suffered a minor back sprain on disability benefits for years while the physicians pursue endless investigations to find "the cause of the pain."

During the 1960s the study of pain gained several new dimensions, which promoted new promising treatment strategies. In the early 1960s, Basmajian (1963) demonstrated that motor units in the muscles can be consciously controlled and changes in function obtained through learning techniques. Years later Miller (1969) and others showed that autonomic visceral and glandular functions can also be changed through training and learning. The foundation was thus set for biofeedback therapy, one of the most useful techniques for noninvasive and nonpharmacological control of pain. In 1965 Melzack and Wall published their famous article on "pain mechanisms," in which they proposed the well-known "gate theory of pain." The gate theory was later proved incorrect in its neurophysiological details but it provided new insights into the discriminative, affective, and cognitive aspects of the painful experience and stimulated further basic research into the neurophysiology of nociception. A crucial state in the evolution of pain treatment followed the pioneering work of Fordyce and his colleagues (1968), when the role of conditioning in problems of chronic pain was demonstrated by effecting changes in chronic sufferers through behavior modification. A new definition was proposed: *pain behavior*—an illness behavior where pain complaints are predominant. Once research proved that learning processes deeply influence the pain experience, a whole new approach to pain management came into practice: the concept of pain control through rehabilitation based on techniques for behavior modification, the so-called "pain clinic approach."

Actually, the idea of specialized medical units devoted primarily to the diagnosis and treatment of chronic pain is not only the product of the research findings of the sixties. It was proposed in the early 1950s by John Bonica (1953) in his now famous textbook, *The Management of Pain*. In this book, which is a classic in medicine, Bonica laid down a clear picture of what pain is and how it should be managed. In 1953 Bonica could not anticipate the findings of the late 1960s, yet he properly stressed the role of emotions in influencing the painful experience. Many chapters of his book are still valid today, even though written 30 years ago. The concept of multidisciplinary pain teamwork, which was almost ignored during the fifties, except for a few pioneers in the United States and elsewhere, became the source of much thinking, research, and clinical application in the 1970s and up to the present. The aggressive surge of interest in pain problems both for research and clinical practice was sparked by a historic meeting of the world's "pain experts" in Seattle, Washington, in 1973, when the foundations were laid for an International Association for the Study of Pain (IASP). The IASP was incorporated in 1974 and held its first congress in 1975—the largest meeting ever held of professionals with common interests in pain issues. Some 1100 registrants from 35 countries and 75 different disciplines attended. The success was duplicated and enlarged during the second IASP congress in Montreal, Canada, in 1978. National branches of the IASP were founded in many countries of the world; the American Pain Society (APS) was founded and held its first meeting in 1979.

Focus on chronic pain has been sharpened in recent years through courses and conferences in continuing medical education, regional and national symposia, audiovisual programs, and good press coverage. In 1976 a report in *Medical World News* listed only 17 pain clinics in the United States; in 1978 the *Pain Clinic Directory* published by the American Society of Anesthesiologists listed over 200 pain clinics and pain control centers, and 285 pain control facilities were listed in the 1979 directory. The growth of pain control facilities obviously responds to a real and urgent need as the enormous cost of chronic pain and the waste in human resources clearly indicate, at least in this country.

PAIN CONTROL FACILITIES

Definitions

Pain

The Subcommittee on Taxonomy of the IASP has proposed the following definition of pain: "An unpleasant sensory and emotional experience associated with the actual or potential tissue damage, or described in terms of such damage."

Algology

This is the art and science of pain management (from the Greek *algos* = pain and *logos* = study, topic).

Pain clinic

A pain clinic is a medical facility for the diagnosis and treatment of chronic pain states. It may use all treatment modalities and accept all pain syndromes, or may use only a few of them and treat only specific pain syndromes. It provides clinical service only.

Pain control center

This center is a medical facility for the management of all pain syndromes with the use of all therapeutic modalities. It offers clinical service and educational programs in algology, and both outpatient and inpatient services.

Comprehensive pain control center

This center offers the same services as the pain control center plus research facilities and other facilities for vocational assessment and counseling.

Goals

The goals of pain control facilities are to provide clinical services for patients with chronic pain, counseling services to the community for prevention and handling of difficult pain problems, and service in the management of pain-related problems of drug misuse. They also seek to cooperate with the legal professionals in settling controversial cases of pain-related disability, and to develop educational programs for discussion and exchange of information on issues of pain and research projects for clinical and basic studies on pain.

Professional Staff

The pain team (Fig. 2-1) consists of (1) physician-algologists, psychologists, and therapists; and (2) core consultants—internists, orthopedic surgeons, neurosurgeons or neurologists, physiatrists, vocational counselors, or social workers. Core consultants should share with the members of the pain team a common philosophy, a common language, and a common knowledge on basic issues of chronic pain.

Patient Population

Five main groups of patients are likely to be candidates for pain control facilities: (1) patients with pathogenic pain from a well-identified nociceptive stimulation of recent onset (mostly posttraumatic algodystrophies); (2) patients with chronic pain from a nonprogressive, noninvasive tissue pathology, an emotional problem, or both; (3) patients with cancer pain; (4) patients with chronic pain who are habitually misusing medications and have developed physical drug dependency; and (5) pain-disabled patients with disability claims and/or litigation who need comprehensive pain evaluation and vocational-disability assessment.

Treatment Programs

All modalities of treatment should be structured in a step-by-step rehabilitation program leading to self-reliance, return to normal function, and gainful employment; PRN treatment is rarely effective in the management of chronic pain. Target areas of any pain control and rehabilitation program are (1) to detoxify patients when they misuse medications; (2) to decrease their subjective

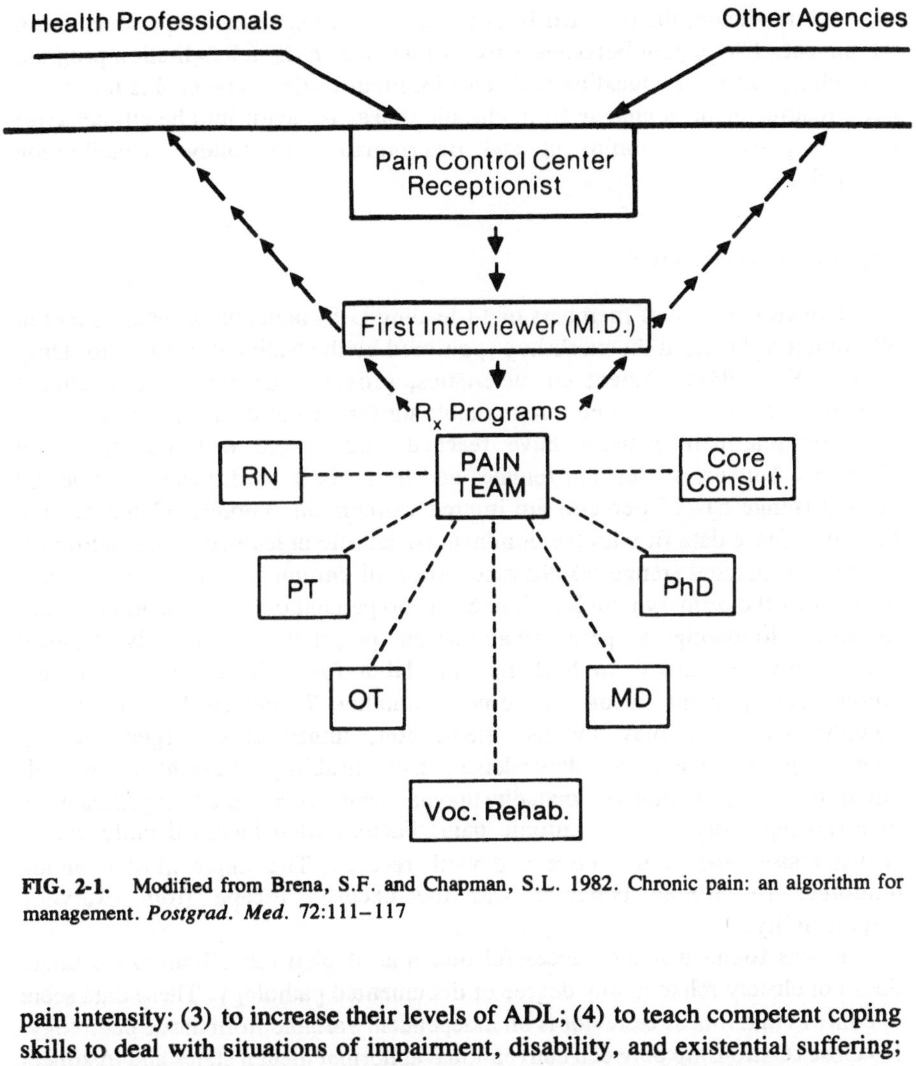

FIG. 2-1. Modified from Brena, S.F. and Chapman, S.L. 1982. Chronic pain: an algorithm for management. *Postgrad. Med.* 72:111–117

pain intensity; (3) to increase their levels of ADL; (4) to teach competent coping skills to deal with situations of impairment, disability, and existential suffering; and (5) to provide vocational evaluation and counseling to pain-disabled patients in order to help them to return to work or other form of productivity.

Patient–Doctor Relationship

In biomedicine the physician is the "knower," the "doer," and the "provider" for a cure of the disease, while the patient is cast into a totally passive role, the recipient of external manipulations, most of them surgery and drugs, with no perceived need for self-commitment and health education. In rehabilitation and behavior medicine, the provider is an educator, sharing his/her experiences with the patient. The patient becomes actively involved in the rehabilitation program through a process of education and behavior modification. The goal is not a cure but a readjustment, a change from chronic illness behavior into health behavior through personal commitment and determination to follow rehabilitation instructions.

Patient Characteristics

Directors and staff members of 14 leading U.S. pain control centers met in Washington, D.C., at the workshop sponsored by the National Institute for Drug Abuse (Ng, 1981). Patient characteristics, program structure, and treatment outcome were compared and a remarkable uniformity of data was found.
Most chronic pain patients have reached middle age with no significant difference between males and females and no specific work pattern. About 60 percent (range 51–77 percent) are injured workers on Workers' Compensation benefits. These data fit with the dominant social role in learned pain syndromes. Around 70 percent (range 50–90 percent) of all chronic sufferers treated show the back as the primary pain location. Some 30 percent of injured workers return to work following a pain rehabilitation program, if properly handled vocationally, to ease them back into the labor force. Ninety percent of the chronic pain patients misuse one drug or another; 70 percent have iatrogenic complications that may include medication, unnecessary surgery, wrong counseling for inactivity, dependence, and disability. Several premorbid, emotional, and cognitive maladjustments were recognized significant in predisposing individuals to chronic pain. Factors cited included child abuse, sexual abuse, and poor service and work records. The single most common reinforcer for illness behavior was the excused escape from everyday responsibility.

It was found that the successful outcome of pain rehabilitation treatment does not closely relate to any degree of documented pathology. These data seem to confirm that illness behavior is an independent variable from tissue pathology. No close relationship between conventional abnormal mental states and treatment outcome was found. The most difficult patients seem to be those who show severe "personality disturbances," that is, chronically manipulative patients with long histories of difficulties in controlling emotions and behavior.

Program Characteristics

No single treatment modality seems predominant in providing long-term improvement in chronic pain patients. Multimodal rehabilitation treatment in parallel was recommended by all the participants at the workshop. The crucial role played by the pain team approach was emphasized. Useful members of a pain team include physical therapists and occupational therapists in an active role as counselors and reinforcers for health behavior. Patients with chronic pain who misuse drugs are usually easy to detoxify since they do not like their drug dependence, which is often iatrogenic.

The program structure should emphasize health education and learning of new coping skills in order effectively to deal with various life stress situations. Most of the pain control programs are inpatient programs. The duration of such programs ranges from two weeks to eight weeks. The cost range is from $4000 to $20,000 for inpatient programs.

Data Collection and Retrieval System

All participants in the Washington workshop recognized that chronic pain is a mammoth national problem of epidemic proportions. They agreed that data must be carefully collected in order accurately to monitor results from pain control programs so that assessments about treatment outcome can be made and results compared. Much research, study, and effort are needed before the epidemic nature of pain can be brought under scientific control. It is imperative that pain control facilities across the country cooperate in providing data from clinical studies of pain patients. Some key questions that need to be answered were identified: assessment of predictive factors from diagnostic work-ups; reliable and valid assessment of results from treatment modalities; identification of factors predisposing human beings to become chronic sufferers; the impact of litigation and disability benefits from conditioned pain behavior; iatrogenic complications from unnecessary surgeries and wrong counseling; and the role of environment in reinforcing illness behaviors.

There are many reasons why pain control units can manage chronic pain patients more effectively and yet less expensively:

1. All features of treatment are performed in one place and at one time, thus reducing the patient's time off the job, travel expenses, etc.
2. Rehabilitation techniques are noninvasive and less expensive than surgical procedures. Most of them can be done without hospitalization.
3. When hospitalization is needed, it requires limited nursing services and no expense for acute medical care such as recovery room and intensive care services.
4. Multiple medical work-ups are kept down by a comprehensive approach to the patient's health problems.
5. Disability cases can be settled promptly when a computerized disability evaluation system is associated with the pain control unit.
6. In a community with a pain clinic, public information about pain is likely to improve, with a resulting decrease in morbidity and disability.

REFERENCES

Basmajian, J.V. 1963. Control and training of individual motor units. *Science* 141:440–441.

Bonica, J.J. 1953. *The Management of Pain*. Philadelphia: Lea & Febiger.

Brena, S.F., Chapman, S.L. and Decker, R. 1981. Chronic pain as a learned experience. In *New Approaches to Treatment of Chronic Pain,* 76–83, L.K.Y. Ng (Ed.) Washington: U.S. Department of Health and Human Services.

Fordyce, W.E., Fowler, R.S., and DeLateur, B. 1968. An application of behavior modification techniques to a problem of chronic pain. *Behav. Res. Therapy*. 6:105–107.

Melzack, R., and Wall, P.D. 1965. Pain mechanisms: A new theory. *Science* 150:971–979.

Miller, N.E. 1969. Learning of visceral and glandular responses. *Science* 163:434–445.

Ng, L.K.Y. 1980. Pain and well-being: A challenge for biomedicine. In *Pain, Discomfort and Humanitarian Care*. L.K.Y. Ng (Ed.). New York: Elsevier/North Holland.

Ng, L.K.Y. 1981. *New Approaches to Treatment of Chronic Pain*. Washington: U.S. Department of Health and Human Services.

3

The Neurophysiology and Taxonomy of Pain

BENJAMIN L. CRUE, JR.

Human pain is better considered as a perception, not a sensation. In acute pain there are often many relationships with both animal and human experimental laboratory pain; but chronic pain in the human in a clinical setting may bear little such relationship. Pain etiology (usually peripheral) must be differentiated from pain mechanism (usually central). Chronic pain may arise within the nervous system from a central generator (repetitive sensory neuronal discharge), with peripheral nociceptive input acting only as either an original etiological or a minor continuing potentiating factor. The existence of premorbid (preinjury or preoperative) predisposing central factors is unproven, but intriguing.

The neurophysiology of pain has emerged from centuries of religious and philosophical dogmatism, inextricably intertwined with religion, mythology, and superstition (Keele, 1957; Brena, 1972). The scientific study of the phenomena of pain originated during the last century with arguments between those advocating specificity theory, such as Johannes Mueller and von Grey, and those suggesting a pattern theory, such as Goldscheider. The organic, pathogenic nature of pain has been emphasized in several monographs (Lewis, 1942; Noordenbos, 1959). One major highlight in the more recent study of the neurophysiology of pain has been the brilliant conceptualization of the gate theory by Melzack and Wall (1965), which postulates a presynaptic mechanism modulating peripheral nociceptive input in the region of the dorsal horn of the spinal cord. Soon after the gate theory was published, other neurophysiologists started to question its true nature, and challenged the sole significance of presynaptic inhibition. The importance of postsynaptic mechanisms was stressed by Crue (1970) and Casey (1973).

The impact of psychological phenomena upon the neurophysiological modulation of the painful experience has seen a resurgence of consideration over the past few decades. Recent contributors in this field have been Merskey and Spear (1967), Melzack (1973), Sternbach (1968, 1978), Carterette and Friedman (1978), and Pinsky (1978).

Acute pain perception is subserved by the sequential activity of various multisynaptic fiber networks from the site of the peripheral injury to the higher brain centers. Peripheral nociceptive transmission involves several structures: (1) *Peripheral "nociceptors"*. These are transducer-like specialized structures and bare nerve endings that have their termination in the skin, in the viscera, and in the deep somatic tissues. Nociceptors have very *high thresholds* to mechanical, thermal, and chemical stimuli, and usually have relatively small receptive fields. Some nociceptors are responsive mainly to mechanical injury (mechanoreceptors), whereas others are responsive to noxious thermal stimuli. "Polymodal nociceptors" may also be activated in tissue damage by several endogenous biochemicals, such as histamine, various kinins, serotonin, and prostaglandins. (2) *Peripheral nociceptive pathways*. Nociceptors are usually considered to be the terminals of a relatively small nerve fiber population, comprising the small myelinated A-delta fibers and the even smaller unmyelinated C-fibers. It has been estimated that approximately 25 percent of A-delta fibers and 50 percent of C-fibers are nociceptors. Other sensory modalities of a more innocuous nature are transmitted by A-alpha-beta fibers. Impulses reaching the dorsal horn of the spinal cord then subsequently undergo a high degree of modulation or sensory processing. (The central mechanisms of nociceptive transmission are reviewed in Chapter 4.)

It must be understood clearly, however, that the newer findings about the nociceptive system may relate only to nociceptive peripheral input from recent injury generating perceptions of acute pain. The role of many higher centers with their presumed interaction with the lower brain-stem system is still largely unknown. The limbic–lobe system (or Papez loop) must undoubtedly play an important contribution through which the higher centers can feed into the hypothalamic area and the medial forebrain bundle for neural and endocrinological interactions and subsequent modulation of peripheral input at lower spinal levels. Recently the work on opiate receptors and the internal opioids has been summarized well by Snyder (1977); it is indeed interesting that the study of opiate receptors involves the limbic system so heavily (Fig. 3-1). Basbaum and Fields were able to publish a model of their conceptualizations regarding a feedback system in their article in 1978 (Fig. 3-2). It is still largely unknown whether there is a direct relation between the opiate receptor system and the various *chronic* pain syndromes observed in humans. (The newer information regarding endogenous opioids is presented in Chapter 4.)

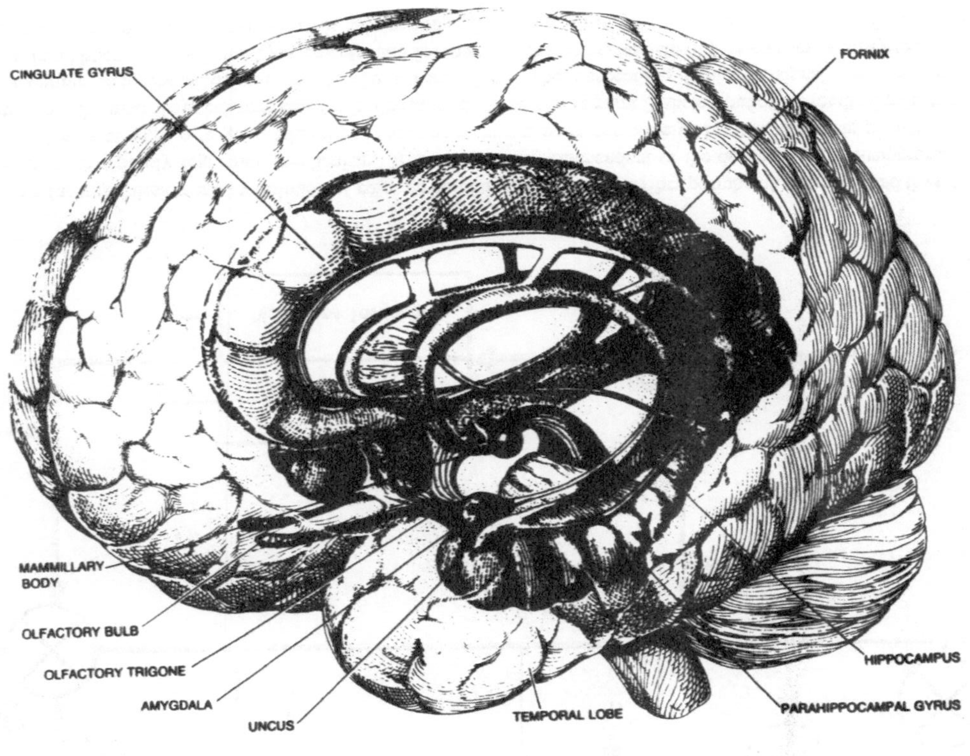

FIG. 3-1. Opiate receptors in the brain were identified by measuring the specific binding of radioactivity-labeled opiate drugs to cell fragments from different brain areas. The largest amount of binding was found in cells from the limbic system (darker), a series of evolutionarily primitive regions at the core of the brain that are primarily involved with smelling in lower vertebrates and with the arousal of emotions in humans. The high concentration of receptors in the limbic system suggests that it is here that opiates exert their euphoria-producing actions, and also that one or more internal opiate-like substances may play some normal role in modifying emotional component of pain (from Snyder, 1977)

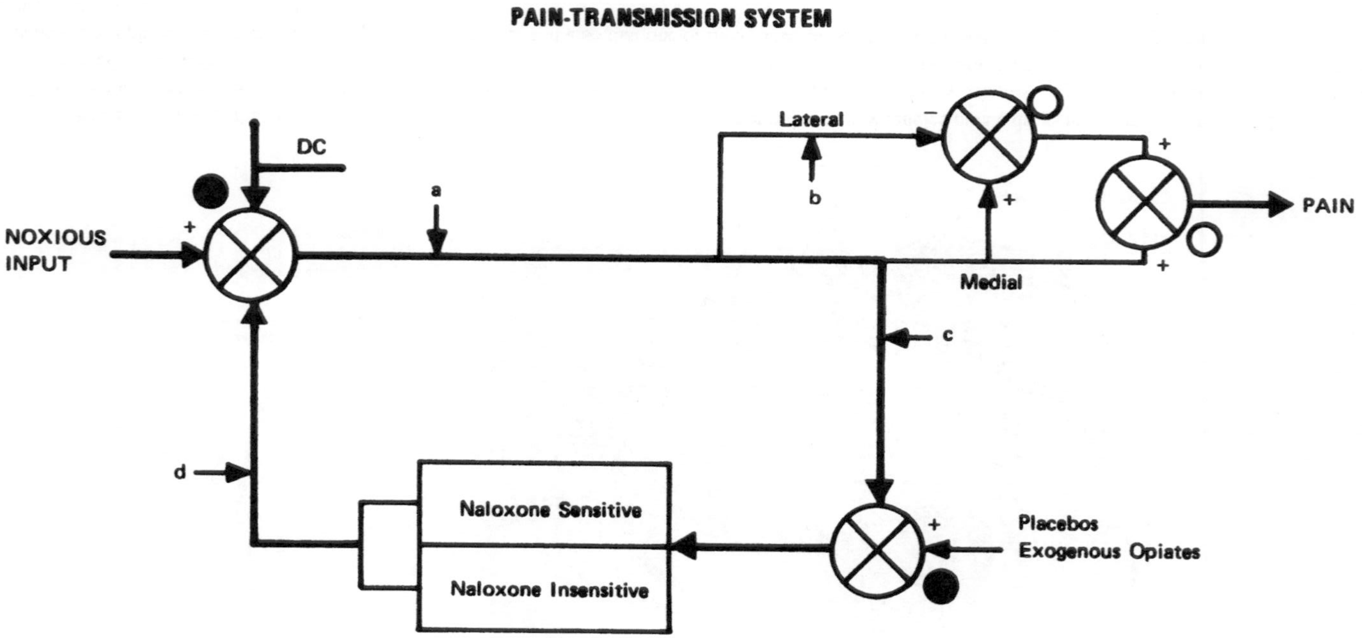

FIG. 3-2. Details of the system for transmission and modulation of pain. At summing point 1, large-fiber peripheral afferents, and thus dorsal column (DC) fibers, inhibit pain-transmission cells through a purely segmental mechanism. This inhibition is independent of the descending pain-suppression system that inhibits the same pain-transmission cells. A lesion at point *a* (e.g., cordotomy) blocks pain transmission completely. Further along the pain-transmission system splits into medial and lateral components. Only the medial system activates the feedback loop. At summing point 2, the output of the medical pain-transmission system interacts with other influences—for example, exogenous opiates or placebo (expectation). The descending feedback signal involves both naloxone-sensitive and naloxone-insensitive pathways. In addition to modulation by segmental and feedback mechanisms, the lateral pain-transmission system inhibits the medial system at point 3, and at point 4 the output of the two transmission systems sum resulting in perception of pain (from Basbaum and Fields, 1978)

PAIN: SENSATION OR CENTRAL PERCEPTION?

One can look at acute pain from the standpoint of neurophysiological *sensation* and consider only the aspect of nociceptive input from the periphery over the sensory spinal and cranial nerves. Or one can consider the way in which sensory information is handled within the central nervous system, and then consider how nociceptive information is processed as it proceeds sequentially cephalad until it is brought to the individual patient's conscious awareness. Such awareness can be considered as the *perception* of pain.

Pain as a perception, however, can be looked at either from the neurophysiological or the psychological standpoint. This dual aspect of the painful perception may create confusion of definitions and cloud the understanding of the phenomenon. A physiological view of the psychology of pain is presently possible, so that some of the confusion can be minimized (Crue, 1975, 1979).

If one considers the phenomenon of pain from the standpoint of the "black box" (Chapter 1) and relates this accepted model to the neurophysiology of pain, the stimulus input can usually be considered to be strictly within the neurophysiological domain. Integration within the black box can be considered as either central nervous system neurophysiology, which is only beginning to be understood in molecular-mechanistic terms, or perhaps it can be better understood and communicated by resorting to psychological terminology. Responsive pain behaviors would then belong in the realm of behavioristic psychology.

Another problem in the neurophysiological study of pain relates to the confusion between "etiology" and "mechanism". Most acute pain has tissue damage as its underlying etiological cause. However, the mechanism of transduction from the area of tissue injury into sequential and probably repetitive nerve impulses generated peripherally and then passed centripetally into the spinal and cranial nervous structures is little understood; still more obscure (even in acute pain, let alone in chronic pain) is the mechanism by which the peripheral nociceptive input is modulated and integrated within the central nervous system to become the conscious percept of pain.

PROBLEMS OF TAXONOMY

Disregarding any consideration of etiology or mechanism, it is possible to reach a useful, though very limited, classification of pain syndromes based only on the temporal factor of duration alone (Crue, 1979). This temporal distinction is an important consideration for understanding the neurophysiology of pain. Indeed there may be little relation between acute pain from tissue damage with nociception and the central neuronal activity underlying human chronic pain.

Table 3-1
Taxonomy of Pain Based Mainly on Temporal Aspect

1.	Acute (up to a few days) (due to nociceptive input from recent tissue damage in most instances)
2.	Subacute (few days to a few weeks)
3.	Recurrent acute (rheumatoid and osteoarthritis, migraine)
4.	"Ongoing" pain in patients with underlying malignant disease—with presumed continued nociceptive input
5.	Chronic (more than six months) benign (nonneoplastic) intractable pain, but where the patient is apparently coping adequately
6.	Chronic intractable benign pain syndrome (CIBPS), with poor coping by the patient

Table 3-1 shows a taxonomy of pain that is mainly based on temporal aspects:

1. *Acute pain*. This definition includes the typical peripheral tissue injury as an etiological agent. From the injured region nociceptive input is generated, creating the subsequent painful perception; such perception will continue until such time as the wound heals, unless the nociceptive input is blocked by a local anesthetic or altered by the use of peripheral and central analgesic drugs. From a neurophysiological standpoint, the healing of the injury, or the removal of the peripheral etiological agent (such as a ureteral calculus), may be expected to end the acute painful perception by stopping the nociceptive input.

2. *Subacute pain*. Clinically this syndrome is based only on the length of time elapsed since the symptom occurred. It is usually taken to be from a few days to a few weeks. From a neurophysiological point of view, subacute pain is quite similar to acute pain in its etiological and nociceptive mechanisms.

3. *Recurrent acute pain*. The predominant etiology of this syndrome is the recurrent acute flare-up of peripheral tissue pathology due to an underlying chronic pathological entity. Examples of recurrent acute pain may include recurrent attacks of rheumatoid arthritis, recurrent radicular pain in patients with hypertrophic osteoarthritis, or degenerative disk and joint disease. It also may include syndromes where the etiology is often unknown, such as classical migraines and trigeminal neuralgia.

4. *Ongoing cancer pain*. Cancer pain may be considered a form of recurrent acute pain with a usually relentlessly progressive underlying pathological etiology and mechanism. Mechanisms of cancer pain are presumably due to inceasing peripheral pathology, as invasive tumor cells cause further peripheral tissue damage and perhaps invade the perineurium of peripheral nerves or plexi. Cancer pain can be well controlled by interrupting nociceptive input (either by peripheral nerve blocks or by neurosurgical procedures) and by altering the

painful experience with central analgesic drugs in doses and time schedules adequate to provide effective analgesic protection (Chapter 12).

5. *Chronic intractable benign pain with adequate patient coping*. The association between ongoing peripheral pathology with intermittent nociceptive input and potentiating central nervous system factors, such as emotional maladjustment, anxiety, or depression, may cause some degree of constant, continuous pain. However, some patients with chronic, intractable, benign pain are able to cope with their continuous unpleasant perception, and manage to live productive lives.

6. *Chronic intractable benign pain syndrome, (CIBPS) with poor patient coping*. When coping mechanisms break down, patients may become completely disabled by the chronic suffering experience, regardless of the originating etiological cause that started the pain problem. These are the "end-of-the-road" pain patients, and are often the victims of multiple, unsuccessful nerve blocks, surgical interventions for pain, and multiple drug misuse (Pinsky, 1978).

PERIPHERALIST VERSUS CENTRALIST

Additional medical intervention aimed at stopping any presumed continued peripheral nociceptive input is usually clinically ineffective in patients with CIBPS, whether or not the etiological cause is known. Even if temporary relief is achieved by surgery or isolated nerve blocks, it usually does not last long, and there is a high rate of recidivism with recurrence of pain and suffering.

At present there are at least two contending schools of thought regarding pain mechanisms, which are reflected in sharp differences in approaching patients with chronic benign pain.

The *centralist* position questions the need for any presumed continued peripheral input (either specifically nociceptive along the A-delta or C-fibers, or as part of a patterned total peripheral input) as an explanation for the continued painful experience. There is no question that some relatively rare pain syndromes may originate entirely within the central nervous system, such as the poststroke central pain in the Dejerine–Roussy thalamic syndrome, or in patients with a Wallenberg syndrome following an infarct in the lower brain stem. There is also no question that in many central organic pathological syndromes, nonnociceptive sensations, such as light pressure, touch, and light heat can be perverted within the central nervous system and trigger paroxysms of acute pain, mostly along the distribution of peripheral nerves, which can in no way be ascribed to continuing peripheral input. A good example of such sensory conversion is tic douloureux (primary trigeminal neuralgia), where light touch on the face can trigger the paroxysms of severe jabs of pain along the peripheral distribution of the trigeminal nerve. Research findings accumulated over the last ten years demonstrate that the mechanism of such neuralgic pain can be best considered as a form of central "sensory epilepsy" in spite of any probable peripheral etiology (Crue, 1970).

Even in acute pathogenic pain, the neurophysiological mechanism is largely central. The specific nociceptive C-fiber and A-delta fibers input system constitutes only a small part of an overall patterning of input, where the addition of both peripheral and central spatial overlapped factors (convergence), temporal factors (summation), and amplitude factors (intensity) give rise to a central "readout," the percept of pain. In humans this readout phenomenon probably begins in the region of the dorsal horn of the spinal cord, and very likely subserves both acute and chronic pain experiences (Crue, 1975, 1979).

The *peripheralist* considers chronic pain within the acute medical models as due to continued nociceptive input from a presumed continuing peripheral pathology. For some hypothetical reasons, the original pathological injury or pathological condition has failed to heal properly, or has not been repaired adequately by the surgeon; therefore there is a continued presumed abnormal input from "the scar." Quite properly it follows that therapy should be centered around attempts to "block" or "cut" the assumed peripheral input.

It is quite likely that in any given pain problem, both peripheral and central neurophysiological mechanisms are involved; thus it is often impossible to make an evaluation and an exact apportionment at any given time as to which is the most important mechanism in any one case of individual suffering. Most physicians and many physiologists appear to be strongly adherent to the classical position that considers pain to be "real" from an organic cause; such strong beliefs are prone to overlook or even disregard the "psychogenic" (or central) aspects of the overall painful experience.

CENTRAL PREDISPOSITION

If the experience of chronic pain is considered predominantly central with some central neurophysiological "generator" being implicated, the next logical question should be, "What conditions within the black box predispose the central nervous system to signal the readout of pain to consciousness, both to initiate and to perpetuate the human suffering?" It is possible that any individual could develop a chronic pain syndrome from sensory overload if the peripheral input were extensive enough and continued long enough to reach a hypothetical, psychological breaking point or to generate a central hyperactive neuronal mechanism for the continued readout of the percept of pain. On the basis of clinical and historical observation, however, it seems that the central factor in the form of a preexisting abnormality is necessary for the development of chronic continued pain.

Table 3-2
Chronic Pain—Predisposing Central Factors

1. Organic lesion within central nervous system:
   a. Pathological (example, poststroke)
   b. Physiological from abnormal peripheral input (example, causalgia)
   c. Combination of 1a and 1b (possible example, tic douloureux)
2. Possible "genetic" inherited defects, or at least individual differences
3. "Functional" environmental factors from physiologically normal but psychologically often "abnormal" peripheral input from external milieu
   a. Past input into memory storage including early nurturance
   b. Reactive factors to acute pain (as often the etiological trigger)
   c. Combination of 3a and 3b (the CIBPS syndrome)

Table 3-2 shows some possible predisposing central factors for chronic pain:

1. *Organic lesion within the central nervous system itself (the brain or the spinal cord).* Various lesions may play the role of central generators: (a) a pathological structural abnormality (such as in some cases of stroke or multiple sclerosis); (b) a neurophysiological central abnormality, secondary to a peripheral etiology, such as nerve injury in causalgia; (c) a combination of the foregoing mechanisms. A likely good example of such a combination is the painful syndrome of trigeminal neuralgia. In true tic douloureux, there probably is a central "neuron" dropout due to aging or vascular disease that possibly combines with some type of peripheral pathology, such as dental disease or abnormal vessel pulsation against a sensory nerve tract or root. This pathological abnormality acts as an organic initiating etiological event, leading to central pain through the well-recognized process of deafferentiation hypersensitivity," with repetitive uncontrolled firing (sensory epilepsy). The hypersensitive central neuronal network, or internuncial pool, then also reacts abnormally by signaling pain in response to subsequent nonnociceptive peripheral input, as mentioned earlier. There is little doubt that the central neuronal networks involved in neuralgic jabbing pain referred to the periphery are probably closer to the primary afferent endings in the spinal cord. In constant chronic pain, more central neuronal networks are likely to be involved; these internuncial pools are probably located nearer the brain-stem core and possibly the limbic lobe (Crue, 1970, 1975, 1979).

2. *Possible "genetic" inherited defects, or at least individual abnormalities.* The second possible predisposing factor to chronic pain syndromes is the admitted probability of genetically determined individual differences in organic brain structure or chemistry. An example of such a possible defect is found conversely in patients with congenital insensitivity to pain.

3. *Environmental factors from physiologically normal but psychologically "abnormal" peripheral input from external milieu*. The third theoretical central factor in chronic pain, mostly in CIBPS, is the possible previous environmental programming within the memory core of the individual sufferer, which will make the central nervous system prone to develop a continuing memory-like painful experience. Such a mechanism does not necessarily require an actual central focus of abnormality in the pathological or even the neurophysiological sense. Factors involved in the pain programming may include: (a) maladaptive learning (possibly to be included under the term "psychological set" of the individual) preexisting the acute pain at the onset of the CIBPS from the initiating etiological peripheral injury; (b) psychodynamic reactive mechanisms following distress associated with acute injury or disease; (c) a combination of the foregoing factors. In cases of CIBPS, any continued input potentiating the painful experience may not be primarily nociceptive, but may even be symbolic. It may also function mainly or entirely at the unconscious level. It may also well arise from within the stored memory of the human computer itself, when triggered by stimuli from either the external milieu or internally.

CONCLUSIONS

The difference between acute pain from peripheral nociceptive stimulation and chronic benign pain from a central generator must always be kept in mind when discussing any aspect of human clinical pain, even from the perspective of neurophysiology. The concept that patients with chronic pain are somehow different, with possibly a premorbid set of pain-prone personality traits, is a highly emotionally charged and often unacceptable idea for many patients and health professionals, both of them trained to the expectation that pain can be "fixed." It takes time and effort to bring patients and their physicians to understand the role of emotions in subserving the painful experience through the unconscious working of the limbic system.

However, in this very concept of chronic pain as a centrally generated experience stands the best hope for amelioration of the individual sufferer. Enlightened psychotherapeutic attempts and learning techniques within a caring, supportive medical setting for utilizing visual, verbal, and symbolic input may enable the patient to "reprogram the central memory banks of the living computer" (the patient's own central nervous system). In this way the individual sufferer can be trained to "turn off" the suffering, or at least to regain adequate coping skills to lead a productive life in spite of any residual pain.

Editors' note: In this chapter the author presents a classification of pain states based on temporal factors. In other chapters pain syndromes are presented according to the presumed prevalent causative mechanism.

Pathogenic pain from dominant peripheral nociception would be equivalent to the classes of acute, subacute, and recurrent acute pain and ongoing cancer pain of Crue; *learned pain* from dominant emotional and environmental factors would fit the picture of the CIBPS of Crue. Patients with chronic intractable benign pain are categorized into two subgroups: Those with adaptive coping skills are likely to be the same described as Class 2 pain patients of the Emory Pain Estimate Model (Chapter 10) whereas patients with inadequate coping behavior (CIBPS) are the same as those described by Classes 1 and 3 of the Pain Estimate Model.

REFERENCES

Basbaum, A.I., and Fields, H.L. 1978. Endogenous pain control mechanisms: Review and hypothesis. *Ann. Neurol.* 4:451–462.

Brena, S.F. 1972. *Pain and Religion*. Springfield, Ill.: Charles C Thomas.

Carterette, E.C., and Friedman, M.P. 1978. *Handbook of Perception: Feeling and Hurting*, vol. V1B. New York: Academic Press.

Casey, K.L. 1973. Pain: A current view of neural mechanisms. *Am. Sci.* 61:194–200.

Crue, B.L. (Ed.) 1970. *Pain and Suffering: Selected Aspects*. Springfield, Ill.: Charles C Thomas.

Crue, B.L. (Ed.) 1975. *Pain: Research and Treatment*. New York: Academic Press.

Crue, B.L. (Ed.) 1979. *Chronic Pain: Further Observations from City of Hope National Medical Center*. New York: Spectrum.

Keele, K.D. 1957. *Anatomies of Pain*. Oxford: Blackwell.

Kerr, F.W.L. 1975. Neuroanatomical substrates of nociception in the spinal cord. *Pain* 1:325–356.

Lewis, T. 1942. *Pain*. New York: Macmillan.

Melzack, R. 1973. *The Puzzle of Pain*. New York: Basic Books.

Merskey, H., and Spear, F.G. 1967. *Pain: Psychological and Psychiatric Aspects*. London: Bailliere.

Mines, S. 1974. *The Conquest of Pain*. New York: Grossett & Dunlap.

Noordenbos, W. 1959. *Pain*. Amsterdam: Elsevier.

Pinsky, J.J. 1978. Chronic intractable benign pain: A syndrome and its treatment with intensive short-term group psychotherapy. *J. Human Stress* 4:17–21.

Pinsky, J.J., Crue, B.L., and Agnew, D.C. (in press). *The Psychology of the Intractable Benign Pain Syndrome*. New York: Spectrum.

Snyder, S.H. 1977. Opiate receptors and internal opiates. *Sci. Am.* 236:44–56.

Sternbach, R.A. 1968. *Pain: A Psychophysiological Analysis*. New York: Academic Press.

Sternbach, R.A. 1974. *Pain Patients: Traits and Treatment*. New York: Academic Press.

Sternbach, R.A. (Ed.) 1978. *The Psychology of Pain*. New York: Raven Press.

Weisenberg, M. (Ed.) 1975. *Pain: Clinical and Experimental Perspectives*. St. Louis: C.V. Mosby

4

Endogenous Opioid Peptides and the Control of Pain

KENNETH V. ANDERSON

The anatomy, physiology, and pharmacology of an intrinsic neural network that monitors and modulates the activity of pain-transmitting neurons is reviewed. This system can be activated by opiate administration or by electrical stimulation of discrete brain-stem sites. Evidence is presented that its pain-suppressing action is mediated, at least in part, by endogenous opiate-like compounds (endorphins). The pain-suppression system is organized at four levels of the neuraxis: the cerebral cortex, midbrain, medulla, and spinal cord. Cortical and medullary neurons project to and inhibit the firing of trigeminal and spinal pain/transmission neurons. Medullary neurons (some of which are sertonergic) can be activated by neurons located in the midbrain periaqueductal gray matter. It would appear that pain itself is an important factor in activating the corticofugal pain-suppression system.

The management of human pain remains one of the most perplexing problems in the field of clinical medicine. Nevertheless substantial progress has been made in our understanding of the neurological substrates that form the basis for the perception of and reaction to pain. One of the most important discoveries in the field of nociception in recent years relates to the finding that there appears to be an endogenous system for analgesia (or antinociception) whose action apparently is mediated by brain substances with the pharmacological properties of morphine. Thus it would appear that the central nervous system itself is capable of modulating sensory transmission in ascending, nociceptive systems that form the basis for painful experiences.

ANATOMY AND PHYSIOLOGY OF PAIN-CONTROL SYSTEMS

To appreciate the central nervous system mechanisms that play an important role in modulating nociceptive transmission, it is necessary to have a basic understanding of the anatomical organization of mammalian nociceptive systems. Fig. 4-1 shows the principal features of the ascending and descending components of a "typical" mammalian spinal pain system. The figure indicates that main nociceptive information enters lamina 1, 4, 5, and 6 via small-diameter fibers, and is transmitted to higher centers of the central nervous system via two major ascending systems. The more lateral system originates primarily from second-order neurons in lamina 1 of the dorsal gray matter in the spinal cord, which project primarily to the ventrobasal thalamus, which, in turn, projects primarily to the somatosensory cortex. The more medial system originates primarily from second-order neurons located in lamina 4, 5, and 6 of the spinal dorsal gray matter. These latter neurons project widely throughout the brain stem, but have their densest projections to the medullary and pontine reticular formation and to the intralaminar nuclei of the medial thalamus. Projections from thalamic neurons go to the somatosensory cortex and to portions of the frontal cortex. In the neuroscience literature, the more lateral pain-transmission system has been associated with sensory/discrimination functions and the more medial system with affective motivational activities. While this general functional characterization is interesting and should be kept in mind, it should be noted that the distinction may need to be altered as more specific information is known about the anatomical-functional attributes of nociceptive systems. For a comprehensive review of mammalian nociceptive systems the reader is referred to an article by Price and Dubner (1977).

In addition to the ascending portions of the pain pathways, there are important descending (or corticofugal) connections. These descending systems are illustrated in Figure 4-1 by the large cross-hatched arrow. As can be seen in the diagram, some of the descending connections originate in the somatosensory cortex and project directly to lamina 4, 5, and 6 in the spinal cord. Other descending connections originate in cell groups in the ventral and lateral regions of the periaqueductal gray matter in the mesencephalon and project to the nucleus raphe magnus in the medulla oblongata and, to a lesser extent, directly to lamina 4, 5, and 6 in the spinal cord (Mayer & Price, 1976). Neurons in the nucleus raphe magnus project directly to the deeper lamina of the spinal gray matter in the dorsal horn.

It should be noted, as depicted in Figure 4-1, that the cell populations in the periaqueductal gray matter and in the medial portions of the medullary and pontine reticular formation are in an anatomical position to play a role in both the ascending and descending control of sensory transmission of nociceptive information in the central nervous system. As the neuronal populations in the descending pain pathways have been systematically studied and characterized, it has become increasingly clear that the descending system plays a crucial role in determining the extent to which sensory information traveling in the ascending pain pathways is permitted to pass from place to place within the central pain

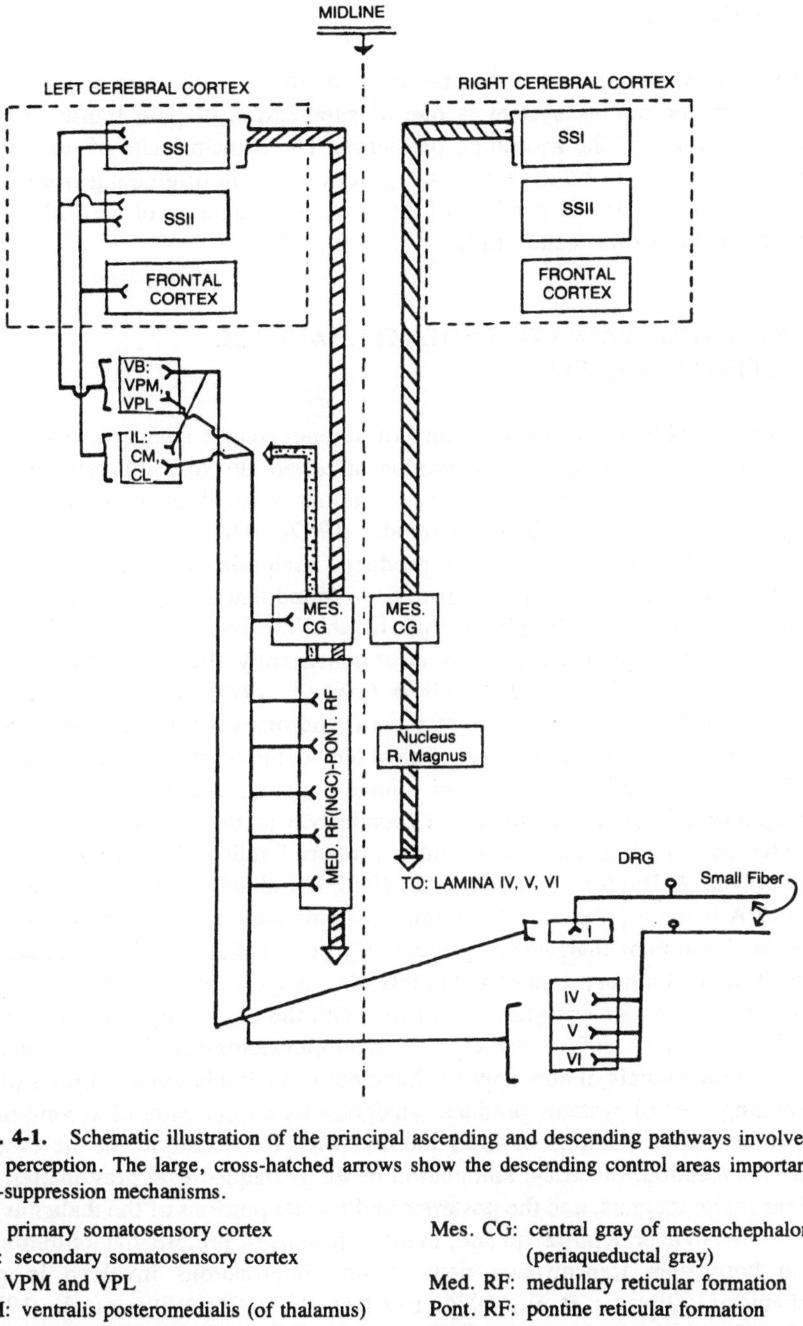

FIG. 4-1. Schematic illustration of the principal ascending and descending pathways involved in pain perception. The large, cross-hatched arrows show the descending control areas important in pain-suppression mechanisms.

SSI: primary somatosensory cortex
SSII: secondary somatosensory cortex
VB: VPM and VPL
VPM: ventralis posteromedialis (of thalamus)
VPL: ventralis posterolateralis (of thalamus)
IL: intralaminar nuclei
CM: centrum medianum (of thalamus)
CL: Centralis lateralis (of thalamus)
Mes. CG: central gray of mesenchephalon (periaqueductal gray)
Med. RF: medullary reticular formation
Pont. RF: pontine reticular formation
NGC: nucleus reticularis gigantocellularis
I,IV,V,VI: Rexed's layers one, four, five, six
DRG: dorsal root ganglion

systems. It would appear that the predominant effect of activating neurons in the descending nociceptive system is one of suppression of pain transmission in sensory portions of the ascending pathways. The principal site of nociceptive suppression seems to be in lamina 4, 5, and 6 for pain originating from spinal regions and in the deeper portions of the descending nucleus of the fifth cranial nerve for pain of oral-facial origin.

ENDOGENOUS PAIN CONTROL MECHANISMS: ELECTROANALGESIA

The earliest evidence for the existence of an endogenous analgesia system was the observation that electrical stimulation of certain discrete brain-stem sites in animals produces profound analgesia, without general upset or depression (Mayer & Liebeskind, 1974; Reynolds, 1969). This phenomenon is now commonly referred to as stimulation-produced analgesia (SPA). Numerous sites within the central nervous system have been found that produce analgesia when stimulated, but electrode placements in the medial thalamus and in the ventrolateral periaqueductal gray are most consistently effective (Kand & Taub, 1975; Long & Hagfors, 1975; Lewis & Gebhart, 1977). The special value of electrically induced analgesia in human pain syndromes became manifest when it was discovered that relief of severe clinical pain could be obtained by stimulating within the central nervous system of human patients. In patients midbrain and diencephalic stimulation at brain sites analogous to those demonstrated to be effective in experimental animals have produced relief of pain from various causes (Long & Hagfors, 1975; Adams, 1976; Hosobuchi et al., 1977). In many ways SPA is more pronounced in human patients than in experimental animals, since the duration of analgesia may exceed the period of stimulation by hours. By contrast, in nonhuman primates and in rats, the analgesia after stimulation is very brief, whereas in cats analgesia terminates with the cessation of stimulation.

On the basis of a variety of neurophysiological investigations in experimental animals, it now appears that electrical stimulation in portions of the descending control systems produces analgesia by suppression of second-order pain transmission neurons or local interneurons. For example, in the case of spinal nociception, electrical stimulation of the periaqueductal gray matter, the nucleus raphe magnus, and the posterior and medial portions of the thalamus has been shown to exert a powerful and, in many instances, preferential inhibition on dorsal horn pain transmission neurons and interneurons involved in pain mechanisms (Oliveras et al., 1974; Beall et al., 1976; Willis et al., 1977). Similar observations have been made at the level of pain-transmission neurons and interneurons in the trigeminal complex (Sessle et al., 1975).

Taken together, then, the electrical stimulation and neurophysiological recording studies clearly indicate that there is a system of descending neurons in mammalian brains that plays a crucial role in modulating nociception. The studies also clearly show that the predominant influence of the endogenous pain-control system is of an inhibitory nature. Left unresolved by the investigations cited thus far is the mechanism by which the corticofugal pain systems exert their inhibitory control over ascending, nociceptive information. While all the answers are certainly not known at this time, it is clear that certain neuropeptides are intimately involved in the antinociceptive effects that are observed after central brain stimulation.

ENDOGENOUS PAIN CONTROL MECHANISMS: NEUROPEPTIDES

The discovery of stereospecific opiate binding sites in the central nervous system constituted one of the most dramatic findings in the recent history of neuroscience. This discovery was quickly followed by studies designed to identify and characterize the chemical properties of the endogenous peptides that are apparently the natural ligands of these opiate receptors. The first endogenous opioids found in the brain and sequenced by Hughes and colleagues (1975a, 1975b) were the pentapeptides methionine- and leucine-enkephalin. Subsequently other longer chain peptides were found in brain and pituitary, and the entire class of opiate-like peptides was given the more generic name "endorphins." On the basis of current evidence, it now appears that there are, in the central nervous system, two independent peptidergic systems. The first is represented by the short-chain peptides, methionine-enkephalin and the leucine analog or leucine-enkephalin, and is spread widely, but unevenly, throughout the brain, spinal cord, and peripheral autonomic nervous system (Kosterlitz, 1979; North, 1979). The second contains the long-chain peptide β-endorphin and is centered around the hypothalamus–pituitary axis, with extensions into the thalamus, midbrain, medulla, and pons.

The general outline of the enkephalin system can be seen in Fig. 4-2. In general enkephalin cells are observed in many nuclei ranging from the spinal cord to the brain stem, including the medulla, pons, and midbrain, to limbic structures, and to the striatum. Of particular interest are the areas with enkephalin fibers and cells potentially associated with the action of plant opiates. For example, the cells in lamina 1, 2, 4, 5, and 6 of the spinal cord in the descending nucleus of the trigeminal system are well positioned for modulating some of the morphine analgesia seen in these structures. Other pain-related enkephalin sites would seem to be the lateral reticular nucleus, the nuclei raphe pontis and raphe magnus, and the periaqueductal gray matter in the mesencephalon. The nucleus

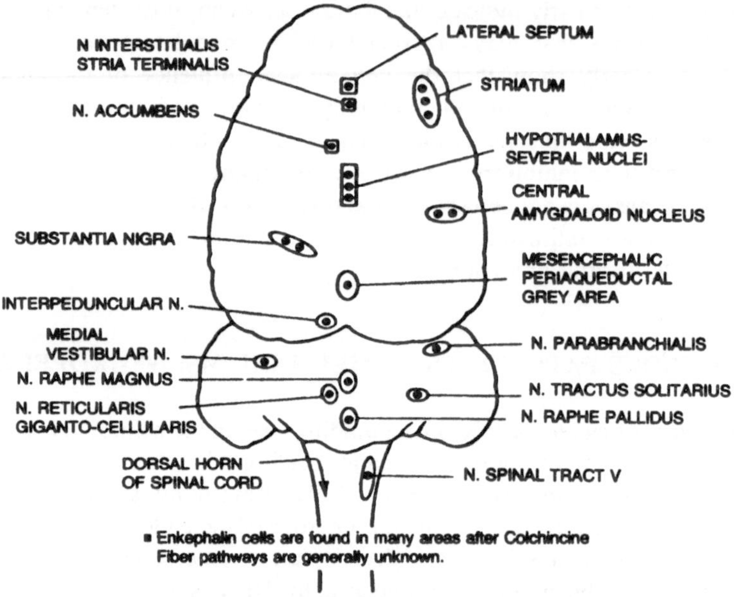

FIG. 4-2. Schematic illustration of a dorsal view of the loci containing enkephalin-positive cells in the rat brain. The illustration is a composite based upon numerous studies utilizing immunocytochemical methods to identify brain regions containing enkephalin

parabrachialis is reported to be involved in respiration and has many enkephalin cells and fibers. More rostrally, in the dorsal-medial aspect of the thalamus, there is a heavy concentration of enkephalin fibers. This general region has been associated with analgesia and opiate addiction and withdrawal.

There are many enkephalin-positive structures in the hypothalamus that are in a position to play a role in certain endocrine functions. Motor systems are also heavily invested with enkephalin-containing neurons. The caudate nuclei seem to contain enkephalin reactive cells and the globus pallidus has extremely dense terminal fields that are enkephalin-positive. Finally, the enkephalins are distributed throughout limbic structures where they might exert strong influences over affective states and moods. For example, there are enkephalin cells in the septum, with fibers near the lateral ventricle, and the nucleus accumbens and the amygdala are heavily invested with enkephalin-containing neurons and fibers. In summary, the distribution of the enkephalins appears to correlate well with those sites in the central nervous system that are known to be influenced by the administration of plant opiates. Of particular importance is the observation that the administration of enkephalins leads to functional changes that are extremely similar to those that follow the administration of plant opiates, including analgesia, respiratory depression, tolerance, endocrine changes, motor effects, and modification of affect.

As in the case of the enkephalins, scientific methods have been developed to help identify the distribution of the long-chain peptide, β-endorphin (β-lipotropin), in the nervous system. Fig. 4-3 shows the general anatomical distribution of β-endorphin-like immunoreactivity in a rat brain. Note that the diagram illustrates a single, major cell group in the periarcuate region of the hypothalamus that has a widespread axonal projection system. The β-endorphin-containing fibers have been visualized primarily in the medial hypothalamus, amygdala, basal septal nuclei, nucleus accumbuns, periventricular thalamus, periaqueductal central gray matter, and locus coeruleus.

While there are minor areas of overlap between the enkephalin and β-endorphin systems, one should note that there are major differences between the two systems. For example, very sparse β-endorphin-like activity has been

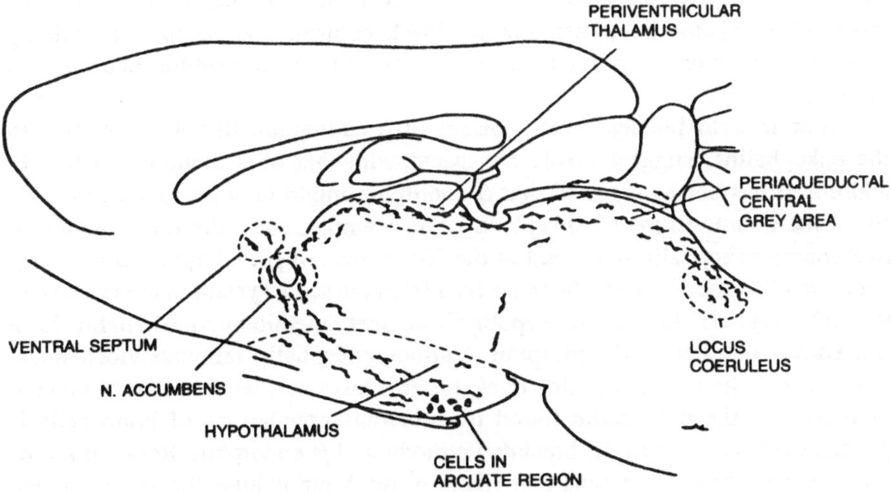

FIG. 4-3. Schematic drawing illustrating a parasagittal view of the rat brain and showing the cell and fiber system containing β-endorphin. Note that the primary cell population of endorphin-containing cells is found in or near the arcuate nucleus and that endorphin-containing fibers are distributed widely throughout the brain stem. Note also that there appears to be an absence of endorphin in the spinal cord

observed in the central amygdala, striatum, and lateral septum whereas enkephalin was seen to be abundant in these areas. On the other hand, β-endorphin-containing cells and fibers were found in abundance in the arcuate region of the hypothalamus, where there were relatively few enkephalin-containing fibers and no major enkephalin cell populations. Thus, at least to date, there is no substantial scientific evidence of cellular overlap between the β-endorphin and enkephalin systems and it would appear that they might function independently and differently.

Taken together the results of numerous immunocytochemical studies of the brain enkephalins and of β-endorphin have led to a variety of interesting conclusions. Based upon investigations of methionin-enkephalin and leucine-enkephalin, it seems clear that these substances are stored as though they were neuromodulators. Their general distribution argues for relatively short pathways, local circuits, and interneuronal functions. They appear well situated for modulation of many of the pharmacological effects of plant opiates. To date no clear difference between methionine-enkephalin and leucine-enkephalin distribution has been identified, in spite of several such efforts. In fact it has been hypothesized that both enkephalinergic forms might be located in the same neurons. If that is the case, then they might be synthesized and released together. It may be that both enkephalins are released from the same neurons, but act on somewhat different subpopulations of receptor sites. If that is true, then the issues of biosynthesis, transmitter feedback control, and receptor specificity become much more complex than in the case of a one-transmitter neurological system.

Immunocytochemical investigations of β-endorphin, like those relating to the enkephalins, suggest a role consistent with that of a neuromodulator. In addition it has been suggested that β-endorphin might be a precursor molecule for at least some forms of enkephalin. For example, since the full structure of methionine-enkephalin is present at the N-terminus of β-endorphin, it has been suggested that they both might be derived from the same system in the brain or in the pituitary. It has been hypothesized that methionine-enkephalin is a breakdown product of β-endorphin. Various enkephalin immunocytochemical studies, including those by Elde et al. (1976), however, would seem to make it unlikely that the enkephalin found in numerous populations of brain cells is generated exclusively as the breakdown product of β-endorphin. Rather it seems that the enkephalinergic cells and fibers in the brain exhibit the synthesis and storage characteristics of neuromodulators, strongly suggesting that enkephalin plays a role as a putative neurotransmitter.

Since the sites from which one can elicit electroanalgesia in experimental animals and humans are also the sites that contain high concentrations of enkephalinergic cells and fibers, it is tempting to presume that electrical stimulation of the nervous system produces analgesia by means of an enkephalin-based mechanism. More generally, it seems reasonable to assume that, together, β-endorphin and the enkephalins are crucially involved in the activation of endogenous, pain-suppressing neurological systems in humans under a variety of conditions, including those occurring naturally and those imposed upon patients during specific courses of treatment. The evidence for the relationship between endogenous opiate-like neuropeptides and the activation of descending control systems that suppress pain is complex and comes from a variety of experimental methods of investigation.

NEUROPEPTIDES AND PAIN SUPPRESSION

The notion that central pain control mechanisms might operate, at least in part, by endogenous neuropeptides produced by the brain and pituitary is based upon several lines of experimental evidence, but the most significant ones are those related to studies in (1) electroanalgesia, (2) the analysis of neuronal responses to nociception, (3) behavioral resonses to pain perception, and (4) acupuncture. Taken together the evidence from these areas of investigation strongly indicates that endogenous opioids play an important role in the activation of descending control systems in the central nervous system that are important in pain suppression. The evidence from these studies also indicates, however, that not all centrally controlled pain suppression depends upon opioid mechanisms. Thus, as is often the case in the fields of medicine and fundamental biological science, the real situation is more complicated than we might like.

Electroanalgesia

As noted earlier in this chapter, there is ample evidence in both animals and humans that electrical stimulation in certain discrete regions of the nervous system can lead to profound analgesia. The sites within the central nervous system that can lead to this stimulation-produced analgesia have been well mapped and in both animals and humans it has been shown the stimulation-produced decrease in pain responsiveness is comparable to that from a large dose of morphine. That endogenous neuropeptides similar to plant opioids are involved in SPA seems highly likely, based upon numerous studies utilizing the opiate antagonists naloxone and naltrexone.

While the evidence has been somewhat conflicting, numerous studies have shown that stimulation-produced analgesia is reversed, or at least partially blocked, by naloxone or naltrexone. Investigations with rats (Akil et al., 1976) and cats (Oliveras et al., 1977) have demonstrated that even profound SPA can be reversed by naloxone under certain conditions. These findings suggest that stimulation-produced analgesia occurs because the stimulation occurs in brain regions that are rich in enkephalins or β-endorphin and results in the release of the endogenous, opioid peptides, thus causing analgesia. This conclusion gains support from SPA studies with humans. The human experiments are most dramatic and show clearly that even intractable pain can be abolished or reduced by electrical stimulation in periventricular and periaqueductal areas of the brain and that this SPA can be reversed by naloxone (Richardson & Akil, 1977; Hosobuchi et al., 1977).

Analysis of Neuronal Responses to Nociception

Within the past few years, an extraordinary number of studies have been designed to evaluate the changes in firing patterns in nociceptors as a function of SPA and the administration of various plant and endogenous opioids. The scientific literature in this area is both vast and complex, but the basic results and technical pitfalls are nicely summarized in a review article by North (1979). In most studies of nociceptors, microelectrodes are used to identify populations of neurons that are either specifically sensitive to nociceptive stimulation, or are at least more sensitive to nociceptive stimuli than to other forms of activation. Single neurons that are especially sensitive to noxious stimuli can be studied to determine the extent to which they can be influenced by electrical stimulation in brain sites known to result in SPA, their sensitivity to opioids, and their responsiveness to specific opioid antagonists.

In general single neurons in ascending pain systems that are particularly sensitive to nociceptive stimuli have been shown to be either completely or partially inhibited during and following electrical stimulation in those areas of the brain that have been described as leading to SPA. These findings would suggest that SPA comes about through the specific inhibition of pain transmission in pathways already identified as playing a crucial role in mediating the perception of and reaction to pain stimuli. The mechanism for this neuronal inhibition would appear to be opioid-related, based upon two lines of evidence. First, it has been shown that many neurons that are especially responsive to nociceptive stimulation are suppressed by both plant opioids and by the endogenous opioids. Second, both stimulation-produced and opioid-induced cellular inhibition can be reversed by nalaxone. Thus it appears that at least some of the alterations in pain perceptions and reactions that occur in animals and humans after electrical stimulation of the brain or the administration of opioids are the direct result of influences exerted on pain transmission neurons by endogenous, pain-control mechanisms. In particular it would seem that the inhibitory influences are operating at the synaptic or, possibly, subsynaptic level.

Behavioral Responses to Pain Perception

As in the case of studies involving electroanalgesia and single-cell neurophysiology, experiments assessing behavioral and perceptual parameters have also implicated endogenous neuropeptides in the control of pain. In many animal experiments, perception and behavior are rigorously controlled through careful manipulation of the environment and the choice of responses. Even the manner in which a response can be exhibited is frequently controlled in a meticulous way. In many types of experiments, using various species of animals, it has been shown that specifically learned responses to nociceptive stimuli can be abolished or radically altered by the administration of enkephalins and β-endorphin. As expected the antinociceptive effect of enkephalins and of β-endorphin have been reversed by naloxone.

In human studies it has been shown that there can be an increase in the amount of opioid peptides in the cerebrospinal fluid after electrical stimulation of brain sites that produce electroanalgesia (Terenius, 1978), and, as noted earlier, Hosobuchi and colleagues (1977) have shown that the pain relief provided patients with intractable pain, after electrical stimulation of the brain, is reversed by naloxone. A recent study by Stacher et al. (1979) considered the effects of the synthetic enkephalin analog FK 33-824 on pain threshold and pain tolerance in humans. The synthetic enkephalin was utilized because it is metabolically more stable than the natural enkephalins and is less susceptible to biological breakdown. In animals, in fact, this synthetic enkephalin has been shown to produce long-lasting analgesia. In humans FK 33-284 was shown to increase the tolerance to pain, but did not alter the perception of pain. Since FK 33-824 and the natural enkephalins do not seem to alter pain thresholds, it would appear that they influence an individual's reactions to pain through mechanisms similar to those that involve the plant opioids.

Acupuncture

A final area of study that provides clues as to the mechanisms by which the central pain systems operate to help suppress nociception is that relating to the use of acupuncture. While acupuncture has long been used by the Chinese to provide a measure of pain relief, only relatively recently has it been used by western physicians. In the United States, a more common technique to produce peripheral electroanalgesia has been that of transcutaneous electrical nerve stimulation. In both animals (Pomeranz et al., 1977) and humans (Mayer et al., 1977), acupuncture analgesia is blocked by naloxone. In the animal experiments, electroacupuncture suppressed the response of spinal cord dorsal horn cells to noxious stimuli presented to the limb, and the analgesia was dependent upon an intact pituitary. Since the naloxone blockade was dramatic and complete, there is the suggestion that, somehow, the acupuncture stimulation caused an enkephalin release in neurons located close to the pain-transmission neurons in the dorsal lamina of the spinal cord (e.g., possibly in substantia gelatinosa). The time course of the effects and the dependence upon an intact pituitary suggest the release, perhaps by secretion back into the cerevroventricular system, of a long-acting peptide such as β-endorphin. It is interesting to note that naloxone has no effect on analgesia induced by hypnosis (Mayer et al., 1977).

CONCLUSIONS

There is ample evidence to indicate that there is, within the brains of mammals, including humans, an intrinsic system of neurons that is involved in modulating sensory transmission in the ascending pain pathways. It would appear that one of the predominant activities of those descending control systems is actively to inhibit the firing of neurons that are especially sensitive to painful stimuli. This active inhibition can be exerted on neurons that are mediating pain of spinal origin or on neurons that are transmitting signals related to oral-facial pain. While it is clear that at least part of this powerful descending pain inhibition depends upon an endogenous opioid mechanism, it would also appear that descending suppression can occur through other mechanisms as well. Interestingly it would appear that the descending pain control systems might be activated by pain itself. That is to say, environmental events that involve tissue damage or produce extreme stress seem entirely capable of activating the endogenous pain-suppression systems, so that an individual's tolerance of and reaction to adverse circumstances can be adjusted.

In spite of what is already known about pain mechanisms, much remains to be understood and numerous questions remain. For example, what specific, natural circumstances cause the release of endogenous enkephalins and endorphin? What specific functional roles does each of the endogenous peptides have? How are their synthesis and metabolism regulated within the central nervous system? How many opiate receptor types might there be within the nervous system? What are their roles in pain control? Finally, since, as far as is known to date, all natural and synthetic opioid peptides are able to produce tolerance and dependence, are humans dependent upon their own endogenous opioid peptides? Fortunately the answer to the last question would seem to be no! The mechanisms that appear to prevent such dependence are the sequestering of the opioid peptides in subcellular structures and the rapid destruction, particularly of the short-chain enkephalins, after their release from the nerve endings. Taken together these factors would seem to limit the duration of exposure of the pharmacological receptors to their ligands, thus avoiding the development of tolerance and dependence (Kosterlitz & Hughes, 1977).

REFERENCES

Adams, J.E. 1976. Naloxone reversal of analgesia produced by brain stimulation in the human. *Pain* 2:161–166.

Akil, H., Mayer, D.J., and Liebeskind, J.C. 1976. Antagonism of stimulation-produced analgesia by naloxone, a narcotic antagonist. *Science* 191:961–962.

Beall, J.E., Martin, R.F., Applebaum, A.E., and Willis, W.D. 1976. Inhibition of primate spinothalamic tract neurons by stimulation in the region of the nucleus raphe magnus. *Brain Res.* 114:328–333.

Elde, R., Hokfelt, T., Johansson O., and Terenius, L. 1976. Immunohistochemical studies using antibodies to leucine-enkephaline: Initial observations on the nervous system of the rat. *Neuroscience* 1:349–351.

Hosobuchi, Y., Adams, J.E., and Linchitz, R. 1977. Pain relief by electrical stimulation of the central grey matter in humans and its reversal by naloxone. *Science* 197:183–186.

Hughes, J. 1975a. Isolation of an endogenous compound from the brain with pharmacological properties similar to morphine. *Brain Res.* 88:295–308.

Hughes, J., Smith, T.W., Kosterlitz, H.W., et al.; 1975b. Identification of two related pentapeptides from the brain with potent opiate agonist activity. Nature 258:577–579.

Kane, K., and Taub, A. 1975. A history of local electrical anesthesia. *Pain* 1:125–138.

Kosterlitz, H.W., and Hughes, J. 1977. Peptides with morphine-like action in the brain. *Br. J. Psychiatr.* 130:298–304.

Kosterlitz, H.W. 1979. Endogenous opioid peptides and the control of pain. *Psychol. Med.* 9:1–4.

Lewis, V.A., and Gebhart, G.F. 1977. Evaluation of the periaqueductal gray (PGA) as a morphine-specific locus of action and examination of morphine-induced and stimulation-produced analgesia at coincident PAG loci. *Brain Res.* 124:283–303.

Long, D.M., and Hagfors, N. 1975. Electrical stimulation in the nervous system: The current status of electrical stimulation of the nervous system for relief of pain. *Pain* 1:109–124.

Mayer, D.J., and Liebeskind, J.C. 1974. Pain reduction by focal electrical stimulation of the brain: An anatomical and behavioral analysis. *Brain Res.* 68:73–93.

Mayer, D.J., and Price, D.D. 1976. Central nervous mechanisms of analgesia. *Pain* 2:379–404.

Mayer, D.J., Price, D.D., and Rafii, A. 1977. Antagonism of acupuncture analgesia in man by the narcotic antagonist naloxone. *Brain Res.* 121:368–372.

North, R.A. 1979. Opiates, opioid peptides and single neurons. *Life Sci.* 24:1527–1546.

Oliveras, J.L., Besson, J.M., Guilbaud, G., and Liebeskind, J.C. 1974. Behavioural and electrophysiological evidence of pain inhibition from midbrain stimulation in the cat. *Exper. Brain Res.* 20:32–34.

Oliveras, J.L., Hosobuchi, Y., Redjemi, F., et al. 1977. Opiate antagonist, naloxone, strongly reduces analgesia induced by stimulation of a raphe nucleus (centralis inferior). *Brain Res.* 120:221–229.

Pomeranz, B., Cheng, R., and Law, P. 1977. Acupuncture reduces electrophysiological and behavioral responses to noxious stimuli: Pituitary is implicated. *Exp. Neurol.* 54:172–178.

Price, D.D., and Dubner, R. 1977. Neurons that subserve the sensory-discriminative aspects of pain. *Pain* 3:307–338.

Reynolds, D.V. 1969. Surgery in the rat during electrical analgesia induced by focal brain stimulation. *Science* 164:444–445.

Richardson, D.E., and Akil, H. 1977. Pain reduction by electrical stimulation in man. I. Acute administration in periaqueductal and periventricular sites. *J. Neurosurg.* 47:178–183.

Sessle, B.J., Dubner, R., Greenwood, L.F., and Lucier, G.E. 1975. Descending influences of periaquaductal gray matter and somatosensory cerebral cortex on neurons in trigeminal brain stem nuclei. *Canad. J. Physiol. Pharmacol.* 54:66–69.

Stacher, G., Bauer, P., Steinringer, H., et al. 1979. Effects of the synthetic enkephalin analogue FK 33-824 on pain threshold and pain tolerance in man. *Pain* 7:159–172.

Terenius, L. 1978. Significance of endorphins in endogenous antinociception. In *Advances in Biochemical Psychopharmacology, 1831–44*, E. Costa and M. Trabucchi (Eds.). New York: Raven Press.

Willis, W.D., Haber, L.H., and Martin, R.F. 1977. Inhibition of spinothalamic tract cells and interneurons by brain stem stimulation in the monkey. *J. Neurophysiol.* 40:968–981.

5

Pain and Emotions

RICHARD H. MORSE

Emotional states and behaviors directly affect physiology and can lead to illness. The theories of classical conditioning, developed by Pavlov, and operant conditioning, developed by Skinner, point to the important role of the environment in shaping behavioral aspects of pain. However, pain also can be a manifestation of difficulties in resolving mutually reinforcing feelings of loss, anger, and depression. Chronic pain patients often turn anger inward and are unable to grieve effectively. Their behavior and dynamics are unique, and thus they require approaches separate from traditional medical or psychiatric patients in diagnosis and in treatment.

EMOTION AND BEHAVIOR

The word "emotion" is derived from the Latin term *ex-motu*, meaning "derived from or expressed through movement." Actually the idea of a feeling expressed through movement was first elaborated by Aristotle, who thought that the heart was the site of all the powers manifested by the mind–soul; consequently the changing motion of the heart accounted for most human feelings, including pain, "the passion of the soul."

Aristotle was not far away from actual human physiology, as interpreted by modern science. Like "pain," "feelings" are an intimate personal experience that belongs to the "black box," the human consciousness. Feelings are overtly manifested through a series of muscular responses, both in the voluntary muscles of the musculoskeletal system (Chapter 7) and in the smooth muscles of the vessels and the visceral organs. "Behavior" can be defined as a set of voluntary and involuntary muscular responses to internal stimuli and to those from the external environment.

Emotions and behaviors only lead to illness when they become maladaptive and cannot be reconverted into coping skills. Well-established studies in neuroanatomy and physiology have indicated the intense influence that emotional states have upon perception and function. It is likely that the descending endorphin system of pain suppression (see Chapter 4) is highly influenced by emotional states. There is every reason to trust that emotional–behavioral management results in physical, constructive change and is part of primary medical treatment.

Nonpsychiatrists, especially primary care physicians, are usually in a superb position to handle the emotional problems of their patients, being masterful in approaching anxiety and "emotional overlay" through the techniques of empathy, reassurance, and ventilation. They also can use behavioral approaches, because such approaches merely represent an extension and systematic arrangement of the familiar emotional sensitivity that they already possess. The physician needs to learn a surprisingly small number of new ideas in order to become a good behaviorist.

BEHAVIORAL FEATURES

Whether we regard chronic pain as an altered perception, a distorted sensation, or an overly learned response, we need to understand the learning or conditioning that underlies the highly manipulative, dependent, and frustrating behavior patterns displayed by patients. Otherwise it becomes impossible for therapists to maintain any objectivity or strategy in their approach to patients or to other members of the treatment team. Pain behaviors can be learned through the processes of classical and operant conditioning described in the following.

Classical Conditioning

When Pavlov, a Russian physiologist, was studying gastric secretion in dogs, he was brilliant enough to reflect upon a fairly simple observation: Stimuli presented at the dogs' feeding time could often evoke salivation, even without the sight or smell of food; for example, hearing the footsteps of the experimenter could suffice. These reflexes or responses occurred under given "conditions" and hence the terms "conditional" or "conditioned reflex" and "conditioned response" were used to describe this process. Let us invent the presence of a solitary hound, Boris. Under ordinary conditions Boris' response to the ringing of a bell is simply exploring or alerting behavior, and his response to food is salivation (Fig. 5-1).

Unconditioned stimulus ——→ evokes ——→ Unconditioned response
BELL ALERTING

FOOD ——→ evokes ——→ SALIVATION

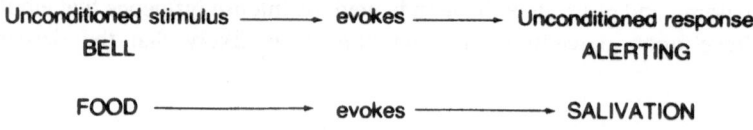

FIG. 5-1. Preconditioning

Now if the unconditioned stimuli are presented together so that food is presented upon the ringing of a bell, Boris will come to pair the bell with the food and will soon salivate upon hearing the bell ring even without sight or sound of food, as indicated in Fig. 5-2.

Thus, through a process of pairing, a neutral stimulus such as a bell can evoke a response such as salivation, which in normal life it would not do. In the life of a chronic pain patient, ordinary, "neutral" objects may evoke pain experience and behavior. For example, most persons associate the sight of their bed with rest, sleep, or other experiences. If the patient's bed has been the refuge sought in the event of a painful experience, the mere sight of the bed may evoke an increase of pain, and also the pain may increase further when the patient goes to bed. It requires but a very few visits to the home of a pain patient to discern a constellation of conditioned stimuli, such as the carefully and mercifully arranged lounging chair in front of the television set beside a small table upon which pills are placed.

There is no doubt spurious story that Pavlov returned home one evening to find Boris happily awaiting him on the doorstep, chewing a bone and freely salivating. Pavlov felt an irresistible urge to ring the doorbell. Such is often the plight of the pain patient's spouse, who responds as if the patient has pain before any pain becomes evident. It is because of such interactions of objects and people with the patient that treatment should begin with a physical separation from such conditioned stimuli as the home and work environment. The family then can be retrained, the environment rearranged, and the patient gradually reexposed to a modified situation.

Operant Conditioning

While the reactions in classical conditioning were referred to a "reflexes" or "involuntary" events, Skinner described another class of responses called "operants," which are emitted by the subject rather than evoked by a stimulus. Operant conditioning refers to the strengthening of these reponses through reward or "reinforcement."

Perhaps the greatest part of our social and emotional learning may be described by the model of operant conditioning. In toilet training, for example, adults shape the child's response to be as close as possible to a chosen desired behavior by using positive reinforcers (such as praise) when progress is made. Undesirable behavior is treated with simple inattention rather than with

Conditioned stimulus ⟶ evokes ⟶ Conditioned response
BELL SALIVATION

FIG. 5-2. After conditioning

punishment. Thus, when a child is throwing a tantrum, an adult can avoid punishing or praising the child, but simply ignore the tantrum while adding positive reinforcement to an alternative behavior such as going out to play. This extinction-reinforcement program is probably the most familiar, humane, and common manner in which healthy behaviors are selected or shaped.

Normal pain, first arising from tissue injury, may be reinforced through its effect on a compassionate and care-taking environment. This contingent reinforcement may persist after tissue damage has largely subsided and may result in "operant pain, or pain maintained by its consequences." The positive reinforcers of operant pain may be deceivingly benign features of the everyday environment: attention from a spouse, the relieving avoidance of work or of unfulfilling sexual experience, and the pleasurable effects of narcotic drugs (long after the analgesic effect has given way to drug tolerance). Simultaneously the punishment of well behavior may occur, decreasing the already compromised remainder of the patients's normal activity . Well-meaning family may "rescue" the patient from healthy activity by, for example, retiring the patient to a sofa and rewarding the growing pain with analgesics.

Classical and operant conditioning are complex and often overlap, as in the case of a pill that is a conditioned stimulus to pain and also a positive reinforcer of pain complaints. In addition the family and treatment team are no less subject to conditioning than the patient, and pain patients can be irresistible in their distress. Further difficulties arise because the patients' homes and work environments are complex and mostly inaccessible to observation and modification. For all these reasons, initial separation of the patient from home and work and constant and continuous training of staff and patients alike are required for successful treatment.

PSYCHODYNAMIC (EMOTIONAL) FEATURES

A commonly shared and central observation was made by Blumer (1975), who concluded after studying chronic pain patients that " . . . it was impossible to make positive diagnoses of known psychopathological categories. The profiles indicated that one probably had to deal with a neurosis but not with any of the known and well-described neurotic reactions." (p. 875). The following cases were recorded because they were so atypical and striking to the medical and nonmedical staff.

Case 1: The Unforgotten Fetus

Mrs. S. was a 45-year-old married woman, for many years a successful career employee of a major governmental organization. After a lumbar discectomy, she was referred to the Pain Unit from a general rehabilitation ward, where the staff had found it completely impossible to bring her from a wheelchair to ambulatory status; electrodiagnostic studies and examination by physical therapy revealed nothing to substantiate this lack of progress.

The patient's husband drove from a neighboring city to attend two interviews at the Pain Unit, which were scheduled about two hours apart. To the amazement of the staff, the couple made an excursion between interviews to visit the gravesite of a fetus stillborn five months into the patient's first pregnancy. The couple had four subsequent progeny, all thriving. The patient returned from the visit in a state of visible grief and agitation.

Observation: Pain patients often fail to display the normal degree and time course of resolution of the loss of a loved object—a person, role, job, physical capacity, etc. As expressed in Fig. 5-3, the normal restitutive sequence of "taking leave" followed by reinvestment of affectional ties becomes blocked.

Case 2: The Angry Lady and the Atrophied Ankle

Mrs. B. was a 53-year-old married woman, a wealthy and highly educated socialite and community leader, who tearfully enumerated the volunteer officerships she had held prior to her disability. Two years previously she suffered a nondislocated ankle fracture and was instructed to abstain from weight-bearing with the assistance of crutches. At her insistence Dilaudid had been used during the acute treatment phase. After 24 months she presented on crutches and consuming Dilaudid, 4 mg every four hours except during sleep. Radiographically her fracture was well healed, but the foot showed extensive decalcification. On gross examination the foot showed trophic changes and exquisite hyperesthesis. The patient's display of pain was massive.

Her husband explained that the patient had always been "spoiled" and that nobody in the family dared breach the myth of her fragile disposition by arguing with her. When the medical director confronted her in group therapy with the observation that she could not admit to the common problem of narcotic addiction plus a disuse syndrome, she accused him of being unprincipled if not delusional, and devoid of any skill or compassion; she announced further that she would certainly "get angry" at him but dared not do so lest her pain should become overwhelming.

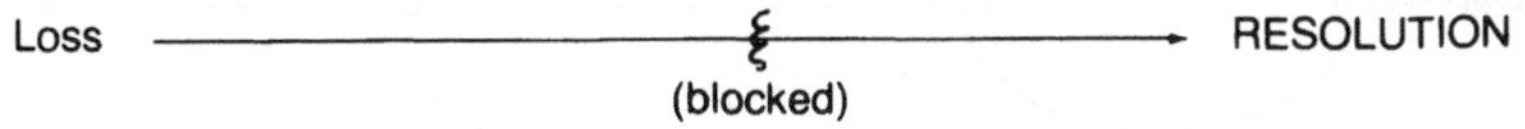

FIG. 5-3. Blocking of resolution of grief

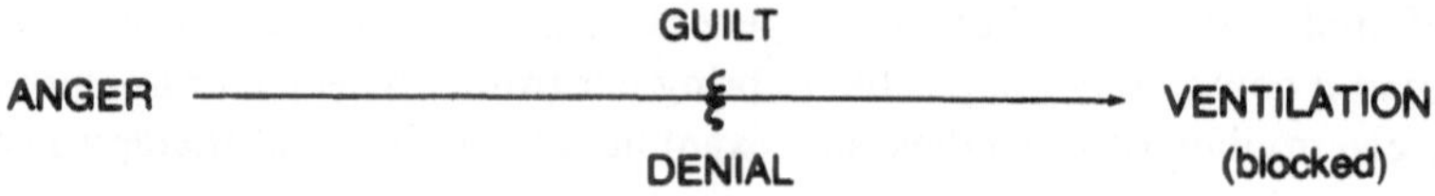

FIG. 5-4. Ventilation of anger is blocked by guilt and denial

Observation: Pain patients often are unable to express anger (and other negative affects) in a usual manner; moreover our culturally strong prohibition against the display of aggression causes such expression to be attended by guilt and denial (Fig. 5-4).

LAD SYNDROME

Throughout their lives normal individuals handle the inevitable losses of important persons and objects without suffering a permanent emotional disequilibrium. Depression and open grieving often accompany such a loss. Sometimes, however, the loss is seen as a desertion and strong feelings of anger are felt. These feelings of anger are often unventilated and are then directed back against the self, thus augmenting depression. Loss, anger, and depression (the LAD syndrome) can become mutually reinforcing unless they are resolved through grief or ventilation (Fig. 5-5).

Because pain-prone patients often are unable to grieve directly and do not ventilate anger because of denial and guilt, they can be left with a powerful set of distressing affects. A vicious cycle of loss, anger, and depression is expressed through pain and becomes the predominant factor in the patient's life (Fig. 5-6).

The somatic pain and accompanying tensions that occur when anger is redirected against the self can be as intense as that experienced with grief or seen in acute pain. To restructure an individual's ability to handle loss is a task beyond most therapies, and certainly beyond the ken of most clinical teams. The two

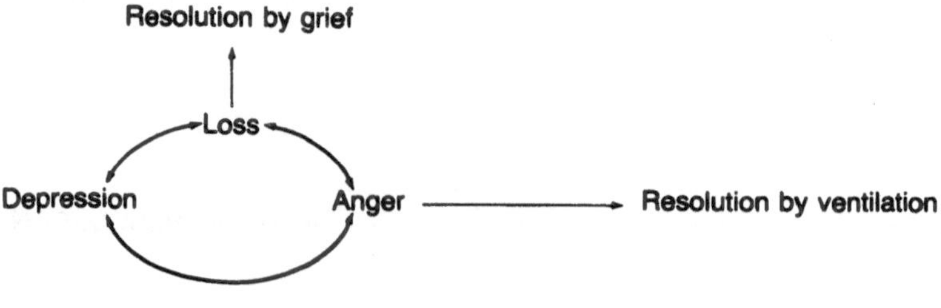

FIG. 5-5. The LAD syndrome

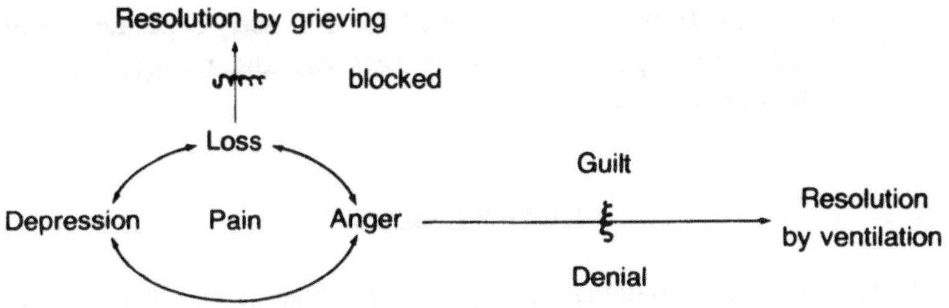

FIG. 5-6. Chronic pain from unresolved loss, anger, and depression

"watchdogs" at the gate of anger,—namely, guilt and denial—present a situation fraught with pitfalls; any simplistic approach to anger, such as encouraging haphazard ventilation through "scream therapy" or other primal techniques, merely provokes guilt and denial, further repressing anger and worsening the whole situation.

The LAD syndrome can be hard to detect through direct observation. Depression and guilt often are not expressed directly during interviews or on psychological questionnaires, since pain patients often have difficulty in recognizing and expressing different emotional states. These problems manifest themselves more clearly in the patients' low self-esteem and demoralization.

Because the patient's pain is a representation of an inability to handle loss, anger, or depression, the patient's actual recovery cannot be measured through verbal pain behavior. Indeed the relationship may be inverse. The more verbal pain behavior is exhibited regardless of its disgruntled content, the less the physiological, nonverbal, or other manifestations of pain. It is often heard from the astute referring physician that the patient had appeared in the physician's office in an angry and verbal manner, debunking all treatment efforts, but had never looked better. Similarly, patients often express ingratitude toward the pain therapist, yet paradoxically are recovering and becoming more independent.

CONCLUSIONS

This discussion of emotional characteristics is a simplified summary of observations by many workers over the years, and the reader is directed to the bibliography to pursue any of the major topics in depth. Despite any superficial resemblance, the chronic pain patient is highly different from cases described as hysterical, hypochondriacal, somatizing, or psychosomatic in character. There is every reason to treat chronic pain patients separately from all other medical, surgical, rehabilitative, and psychiatric patients, both in approach and in physical allocation of facilities. Further, there is need for distinctly separate training and teams and a need for the pain therapist to reassess and reorganize traditional approaches to the patient.

REFERENCES

Blumer, D. 1975. Psychiatric considerations in pain. In *The Spine*, vol. II. R.H. Rothman (Ed.). Philadelphia: W.B. Saunders.

BIBLIOGRAPHY

Bachrach, A.J. 1975. Learning theory. In *Comprehensive Textbook of Psychiatry,* vol. II. A.M. Freedman, H.I. Kaplan, and B.J. Saddock. (Eds.). Baltimore: Williams & Wilkins.

Engel, G.L. 1959. "Psychogenic" pain and the pain-prone patient. *Am J. Med.* 26:899–918.

Fordyce, W.E. 1976. *Behavioral Methods for Chronic Pain and Illness*. St. Louis: C.V. Mosby.

Lindermann, E. 1979. *Beyond Grief*. New York: Aronson Press.

Mahler, M.S. 1979. *The Selected Papers of Margaret S. Mahler*, vol. II. New York: Aronson Press.

Melzack, R. 1973. *The Puzzle of Pain*. New York: Basic Books.

Sifneos, P.E., Apfel-Sasvitz, R., and Frankel, F.H. 1977. The phenomenon of "alexithymia." *Psychother. Psychosomat.* 28:47–57.

6

The Role of Learning in Chronic Pain

STANLEY L. CHAPMAN

The expression of pain depends on an individual's learning history as well as on current environmental influences. Our society and culture begin to shape our attitudes about pain at an early age, and many American values seem to encourage and perpetuate pain complaints. Although cognitions and personality clearly influence pain behaviors, it often becomes difficult to assess whether these factors are precipitating, predisposing, or the results of pain. Pain behavior also can be controlled by its consequences, though the rewards of persistent pain behavior often are quite meager.

Unlike acute pain chronic pain states often are characterized by pain behaviors that cannot be explained on the basis of biomedical findings; two people with the same apparent degree of physical pathology show great divergences in pain behavior. It is tempting to conclude that the differences must be "psychological" or reflect the influences of learning. Because the biological mechanisms and mapping of chronic pain remain unclear, however, this easy conclusion may be unwarranted.

Conclusions about the role of learning in chronic pain should be based on positive findings from relevant assessment rather than on the inability of biomedical findings to account for pain behavior. However, to date there have been no epidemiological studies performed to identify adequately what psychological problems predispose an individual to chronic pain. Rather our attempts to understand the psychology of the pain experience have been based on testing, interviewing, and observing individuals who already are complaining of chronic pain and to compare them with groups of normals. This method contains many pitfalls, including the old cart/horse problem of whether the observed psychological problems predisposed the person to pain, precipitated the pain, and/or resulted from it. In most cases the pain complaints and the person's emotions have become so inextricably intertwined that they are impossible to separate. The question of whether chronic pain is organic or functional loses meaning in view of the way the body and mind constantly interact. The two really cannot be separated at all, as all perceptual experiences have a physiological basis and physical stresses generally have psychological effects.

These difficulties in understanding the mechanisms of chronic pain suggest the importance of assessing carefully a wide range of factors that influence its expression. The importance of learning is suggested by research on social and cultural influences and on the effects of personality and reward on chronic pain behavior.

SOCIAL AND CULTURAL FACTORS

We learn much about who we are and how to respond effectively by observing others in our environment. Starting at birth we begin to learn such things as under what circumstances we should complain about pain, what forms these complaints should take, and what the consequences of such complaints will be. Apley's (1975) study of 1100 British school children over the age of 3 suggests the importance of observational learning in chronic abdominal pain. Apley found that there was a positive family history of abdominal pain in only one eighth of those children whose pain had a clear organic etiology; however, if no organic evidence for the problem could be found, there was a positive family history in fully half the cases. In addition he found five to six times the number of pain complaints in the families of children with abdominal pain as compared with those families of children with no abdominal pain. It appears that many of the children had learned to focus on and complain of pain from observing behavior in their families.

Results from the Kaiser Foundation suggest some reliable differences between different cultural groups regarding willingness to tolerate pain caused by pressure applied to the heel (Woodrow et al., 1972). After studying 41,119 patients, researchers concluded that individuals of English or Irish descent generally were much more likely to "keep a stiff upper lip" in response to the pain stimulus, whereas individuals of southern Mediterranean descent generally tolerated pain less readily. Zborowski's (1969) findings that these ethnic differences in pain expression are most prominent in first-generation immigrants further underscores the importance of social modeling.

Our own society in many ways encourages and perpetuates pain complaints. The values of forbearance and acceptance of pain and medical problems have given way to the attitude that an individual should expect all personal ills to be removed through medical intervention. Chronic pain is seen almost as a denial of a right and an individual is expected to continue complaining and seeking help until that right is restored. Our legal system often compensates individuals for loss of the right through disability grants, and sometimes perpetuates pain behavior in the process.

In our society a distinction is made between physical problems, which are seen largely as beyond an individual's control, and emotional problems, which are stigmatized. (Evidence of this distinction is often seen in professionals who label a pain patient as a "crock" or a malingerer if appropriate physical pathology cannot be found.) Chronic pain patients thus are more likely to gain acceptance and favorable legal settlements if they express difficulties in physical terms and seek medical interventions for documentation or removal of physical pathology. Physicians often are placed in a position in which their only way to please the consuming public is to order extensive medical testing, prescribe habit-forming medications, and/or perform surgeries, all of which can perpetuate pain behavior. There often is no room in the system for the acceptance of limitation and discomfort and the maintenance or reestablishment of maximum physical and psychological function through rehabilitation.

COGNITIVE FACTORS

Recently there has been an increasing appreciation of the influence of learned attitudes and beliefs and of attentional factors on pain complaints. Data from experimental studies in which an acutely painful stimulus of a controlled intensity is provided to a group of volunteers have shown higher ratings of pain tolerance if the subjects expected the stimulus to be painful, believed they had no control over it, or were instructed to attend to it closely (Meichenbaum, 1977).

In clinical pain expectancy and attention often are closely linked with the perceived meaning of the pain experience. Many people have marveled at the tremendous pain tolerance demonstrated by soldiers in battle and by athletes in the midst of competition. Women in some cultures give birth without apparent pain, and members of religious sects who glorify martyrdom or see pain as purifying are able to tolerate normally nociceptive input with little or no evidence of suffering or discomfort. If similar input is perceived in different contexts devoid of positive meaning, it is likely to be experienced or tolerated much differently.

The same variables of expectation, perceived control and meaning, and attention affect the experience of chronic pain continually. For many chronic sufferers, pain is seen as a lifelong companion over which they have no control. Many attend to little else; pain is the central force in their lives and disrupts the social, sexual, recreational, and vocational spheres. The perceived meaning of chronic pain is totally negative; many chronic pain patients see their pain as robbing their lives of any meaning and any pleasure.

PERSONALITY FACTORS

Chronic pain sufferers frequently show evidence of psychological disturbances on personality tests. For example, they frequently show elevations on the scales labeled "Hypochondriasis", "Depression," and "Hysteria" on the well-known Minnesota Multiphasic Personality Inventory (MMPI) and on the "Neuroticism" scale of the Eysenck Personality Inventory given widely in Great Britain. These tests can provide important information about the emotional characteristics of patients; however, because many items on them could be expected to be endorsed by normally well-functioning individuals with serious medical problems, results should be interpreted with utmost caution. Emotional difficulties probably can be conceptualized best as putting a person at a higher risk to develop any of a variety of psychosomatic problems, including chronic pain. How these difficulties are manifested undoubtedly depends on a myraid of somatic characteristics as well as on the individual's unique learning history.

Depression and Learned Helplessness

Chronic pain frequently is associated with symptoms of depression, such as loss of hope and self-esteem, flat affect, low energy levels, inactivity, decreased sexual interest and participation, and disturbances in appetite and sleep. This similarity has led some people to conceptualize chronic pain as a "masked depression," or an expression in physical terms of an underlying depressive state. People from certain cultural backgrounds undoubtedly have learned to express emotional upset in the form of somatic complaints. Moreover it has been found that pain complaints often are lessened with the use of tricyclic antidepressants. On the other hand, many individuals complain of constant and chronic pain while maintaining a high level of activity and self-esteem and without showing evidence of any underlying depressive features. One seldom sees in chronic pain the characteristics of a psychotic or endogenous depression such as a cyclical character, feelings of depersonalization, weight loss, and a family history of depression. Much more frequent is a general feeling of being demoralized.

The theory of learned helplessness developed by Martin Seligman and his colleagues (1975) can account for many of these depressive behaviors frequently seen among chronic pain patients. Seligman found that animals and humans exposed to situations in which their responses could not control outcomes would show three classes of deficits: their motivation would be decreased; they would lose their ability to learn new tasks in which they could control outcomes; and they would show emotional disturbances, chiefly those associated with passivity and helplessness. This syndrome is similar to that observed in many chronic pain sufferers. They appear passive, listless, and helpless, and express little ability to find pleasure or effect positive outcomes in any aspect of their lives. In many cases these individuals present long histories of "helplessness training," characterized by an inability to achieve rewards contingent on their own efforts. In other cases helplessness developed or increased since the onset of their pain complaints. Perhaps they were unable to cope with the stresses and limitations initially brought on by an injury or life event and become more and more dependent on others while losing more and more confidence in their ability to function. These feelings of helplessness may have been exacerbated by a long series of inconclusive medical tests and treatments, dependence on depressant medication, inactivity, and cessation of a productive role in life. Feelings of depression and helplessness must be addressed and treated in any pain rehabilitation program, as a passive person without hope is unlikely to assume the active role required to increase physical and emotional function.

Anxiety

Acute anxiety clearly decreases pain tolerance. When tension or anxiety is prolonged, however, a great number of atypical musculoskeletal, visceral, metabolic, endocrine, and neurological disorders can occur, many of which are associated with chronic pain. The mutually reinforcing effects of increased pain and increased anxiety and tension are underscored by consistent findings that methods that reduce anxiety also reduce pain in the clinical setting. Unfortunately many chronic pain patients are unable to reduce anxiety effectively, and remain unaware of its role in worsening their pain and suffering.

Anxiety is a normal response to changes in life events or to medical problems and is often related to an individual's uncertainty about how well that individual will be able to adapt to them. If the person feels able to gain control satisfactorily over the situation, the anxiety is likely to diminish; if not, the person is likely to attempt to reduce it. One way of doing so is through the afore-described learned helplessness syndrome—to withdraw, stop trying to control one's life, and passively rely on others. The bland focusing on physical complaints seen in many chronic pain patients can help reduce anxiety by providing the individual consciously or unconsciously with a socially acceptable focus for an inadequacy or failure to cope.

THE ROLE OF REWARD

As defined by Richard Morse in Chapter 5, behavior often is controlled by its consequences. If it is followed by reward, it has a high probability of recurring; if it is ignored or followed by punishment, it has a low probability of recurring.

The word "pain" has powerful consequences in our society. The existence of pain is seen as a disruption of every form of human activity, and as a signal of bodily harm and disease; observation of pain behaviors in others often causes great emotional arousal. Pain behavior thus can communicate powerful messages to others, such as "Please take care of me," "I can't do that," or "I need some sympathy." As outlined by Morse, the consequences of such behavior usually include suggestion of rest and inactivity, administration of "pain-relieving" medications, sympathy and attention, and possibly financial compensation. The longer these consequences continue, the more likely it is that the patient will have become inactive, physically weak, or drug dependent, and will feel helpless and useless. Those around the patient also may have altered their life-styles, assumed the role of care givers, and cast that patient in the identity of a chronic sufferer. Even if the original source of pain is no longer present, the process of shifting back to health behaviors may be quite difficult.

In many cases pain behaviors develop or persist not just because they are rewarded, but also because one cannot meet one's needs through alternative health behaviors. The worker who is getting old and no longer feels able to tolerate job-related stresses and responsibilities, the individual unable to find love or social acceptance, the angry spouse unable to express hurt or resentment directly, or the sexually dysfunctional individual unable to deal with sexual problems all might be likely candidates for reliance on pain behavior to avoid stress or to communicate their needs. In these cases pain behavior rarely represents malingering. The sufferer might remain quite unaware that such behavior has been built up and maintained as a result of its consequences.

Pain behavior is just as likely to persist as a result of ignorance as it is as a result of reward. Often neither the sufferer nor the sufferer's family *realizes* that the pain is not a symptom of a progressive disease, that the medications are maintaining depression and dependency, or that physical function could be increased without risk of further harm. One needs to remember that the rewards of persistent pain behavior generally are quite meager compared with those that result from effective well behavior. Disability benefits generally are barely adequate to maintain a subsistence income; depression and dependency often accompany relief from stresses or responsibilities; sympathy and attention from others usually wear thin in a fairly short period of time; and pain behaviors generally prove ineffective ways to solve intraphysic conflicts or to communicate feelings to others.

SUMMARY

In summary a wide range of factors dependent on learning influence pain responses. As indicated in Chapter 3, under certain circumstances input from the environment can become actual nociceptive input in the sense that it disrupts the integration of the "black box" to the point of creating a pain response. These factors can become as upsetting as a heat or mechanical stimulus.

REFERENCES

Apley, J. 1975. *The Child with Abdominal Pains*. Oxford: Blackwell.

Meichenbaum, D. 1977. *Cognitive–Behavior Modification*. New York: Plenum Press.

Seligman, M.E.P. 1975. *Helplessness*. San Francisco: W.H. Freeman.

Woodrow, K.M., Friedman, G.D., Siegelaub, A.B., and Cohen, M.F. 1972. Pain tolerance according to age, sex and race. *Psychosomat. Med.* 34:548–556.

Zborowski, M. 1969. *People in Pain*. San Francisco: Jossey-Bass.

7

Disuse Syndrome: Fibrositic and Degenerative Changes

RENE CAILLIET

Pain of musculoskeletal origin is among the most frequent problems in general practice. Musculoskeletal nociception is enhanced by conditions of disuse and degeneration. These terms are defined. Trigger points with related fibrositic changes in muscles and degenerative changes in articular joints are critically analyzed, with special emphasis on the mechanism of nociceptive stimulation in the degenerative joint disease. Common postural disuse syndromes and the impact of "chronic tension" upon the musculoskeletal system are described.

Pathogenic pain of neuromusculoskeletal origin is among the most frequent problems experienced by the primary practitioner. The musculoskeletal system is a major site of nociceptive stimulation, whose acute manifestations eventually evolve into chronic pain states. These painful conditions are attributed to, or at least reinforced by, disuse and degeneration.

Disuse is defined as "to cease to use" or "cessation of use, practice or exercise" in *Webster's New Twentieth Century Dictionary* (1978).

Degeneration is defined as "to pass from a good to a bad or worse state; to lose former, normal, or high qualities"; in medicine, degeneration is also defined as "biochemical changes in tissues or organs caused by injury and disease and leading to loss of vitality, of function, etc." This simplistic definition, however, does not consider all aspects of degeneration.

Degeneration creates structural changes that feed back additional nociceptive inputs that reinforce the mechanical aspects of disability. Disuse and degeneration are prominent factors of the "five D's" syndrome of learned pain.

FIBROMYOSITIS SYNDROME

Fibromyositis, also known as fibrositis, myofascitis, myogelosis, and psychogenic rheumatism, has been recognized as a specific pathological entity that persists after trauma (Weinberger, 1977). It is accepted as the most common cause of noxious stimulation in the musculoskeletal system and is clinically expressed by tender muscles, nodules, stiffness, and spasm. The diagnosis of fibromyositis is made mostly on reports of pain and clinical findings with little or no laboratory confirmation. Patients do not have fever, leukocytoses, increased sedimentation rate, or alteration of serum enzyme levels. Electromyographic abnormalities have been claimed but none have yet been consistently confirmed (Kraft et al., 1968).

In the absence of organic findings, the pain from fibromyositis has been considered of primary psychophysiological origin, yet the disorder has been unresponsive to psychiatric therapy.

The subjective criteria for the fibrositis syndrome have been summarized as follows (Moldofsky et al, 1975):

1. Subjective aching and stiffness for more than three months
2. Chronic fatigue and poor work tolerance for more than three months
3. Sleep disturbances for more than three months
4. Morning aching and stiffness
4. Weather effect
5. Temporary relief from heat
6. Poor appetite

Many of these symptoms are vague and have psychological implication. Sleep disturbances have been objectively documented by electroencephalogram studies (Smythe & Maldofsky, 1977–78); however, "normal" people caused to have sleep deprivation did not develop fibrositis symptoms. Fibrositic patients treated with chlorpromazine overcame their sleep disturbances and lost their fibrositic symptoms, only to have recurrence of their fibrositic syndromes after discontinuation of the drug. This interesting correlation attributed to the serotonin metabolosm needs further elucidation and verification.

The fibrositic syndrome is characterized by the presence of "trigger points" (Cooper, 1961). The trigger point is a small circumscribed hypersensitive area in muscles or their connective tissues. These trigger zones, when stimulated, frequently produce pain in a distant area (Travell & Rinzler, 1952). The term "trigger" is used to specify that "zone" which, when stimulated, produces a painful perception in a distant "target" area. The exact neurological pathway for this phenomenon is not yet fully understood.

On the assumption that nodules or triggers are of inflammatory nature, injections of an anesthetic agent supplemented by steroids have effectively relieved the muscular pain. However, beneficial results have also been documented following injections of saline (Sola & Kuitert, 1955), or merely dry needling. Extravasation of platelets following trauma releases serotonin with resultant vasoconstriction; the local edema in turn releases mast cells that secrete histamine and heparin (Cailliet, 1977). Swelling results from these various metabolic derangements and may explain the existence of the nodule or trigger zone. The trauma that may initiate this phenomenon may not necessarily be a severe acute injury. In fact it may be a result of a repetitive subminimal traumata of which the patient is unaware and does not remember. This microtrauma may result from postural defects, stress, depression, or fatigue. Intense extremes of temperature, such as intense heat and cold, may also create these triggers.

The trigger area is tender and reveals muscle spasm. Local vasomotor signs such as pallor, sweating, or edema can frequently be elicited. The patterns of trigger and target areas remain constant and predictable, yet do not follow a dermatomal pattern.

Stimulating the trigger area may cause an acute explosive reaction. The referred target zone is usually dull and achy in character; the deep area of hyperalgesia, tenderness, and hyperesthesia of the referred zone may remain long after the trigger irritability has waned. As a result of spasm, ischemia, and metabolic derangements, the referred target zone itself becomes an irritable zone, and this may evolve into a trigger area in its own domain. The ensuing nociceptive cycle becomes chronic and repetitive, and the original etiological factors may not be remembered.

Posture is a common causative factor in creating a myofascial pain syndrome and may be secondary to occupation, fatigue, anxiety, depression, or aging. The most common postural myofascial pain pattern is the so-called "scapulo-costal syndrome" (Michele et al., 1950). In the development of this syndrome, the rounded shoulder posture places the scapula under gravity pull that causes it to rotate laterally. The shoulder girdle, being heavy, places traction upon the levator scapular muscle that attaches to the superior medial angle of the scapula. This point of myofascial periosteal attachment becomes a trigger point. Discomfort is felt locally and is referred to the neck and to the occipital area, causing occipital headaches. By this posture the cervical spine becomes lordotic and causes foraminal closure with nerve root entrapment and consequent radicular pain down to the arm. The downward traction upon the scalenes results in the development of the cervico-thoracic outlet syndrome, with related symptoms in the affected neurovascular bundle.

Another common myofascial syndrome is the so-called "upper trapezius syndrome"; postural strain, fatigue, depression, and prolonged occupational postural stress are common irritating factors. The trapezius trigger zone is usually located in the superior medial border of the muscle or in the intrascapular portion of it. Discomfort is referred to the base of the skull or to the temporal area of the scalp; the neck muscles also become tense and tender.

Patients who develop residual neck, head, or shoulder pain and limitation after a hyperflexion–hyperextension injury, the so-called "whiplash" injury, possibly have a posttraumatic myofascial syndrome. As the immediate result of a deceleration injury, the extensor muscles of the neck undergo a passive unexpected stretch. This sudden elongation of muscle fibers discharges the muscle spindle, initiating a spinal reflex that causes an immediate resultant reflex contraction of that same muscle. This stretch reflex does not occur from a voluntary contraction of that muscle, as there normally are extrapyramidal reflexes that inhibit a stretch reflex and permit an uninhibited muscle contraction. This reflex is not functioning in the acute overwhelming stretch of the muscle. In the whiplash the reflex contraction is essentially proportional to the abruptness and intensity of the stretch force (Bard, 1956). The patient's head is abruptly propelled forward, which imparts an acute stretch on the extensor neck muscles, and these in turn act reflexly to minimize the forward head motion. The violent isometric contracture of the extensor muscles of the neck may result in injury to the muscle fibers. Because only fibers, not large muscle masses, react reflexly, there is no blood vessel injury and no gross edema, and there is no immediate painful perception. However, a myofascitis with local pain, tenderness, and limitation of motion develops within hours or days after the injury (Brendstrup et al., 1957).

Similar acute stress occurs to the neck flexors as the neck is propelled backward from a rear-end collision. This creates a trigger area in the sternocleidomastoid muscles and the short-neck flexors. The referred target zone of this trigger area has been mapped as ipsilateral frontalis and temporal area with a residual headache to be expected. The prevertebral fascia is also damaged from this injury. As the greater occipital nerve passes through this deep cervical fascia, it becomes irritated and contributes to the headache syndrome. Long after the acute injury has healed, the neurological symptoms can persist.

The diagnosis of a myofascial syndrome depends upon finding a tender area which, when stimulated, reproduces the specific local discomfort and/or the referred target pain. To confirm the diagnosis, the painful perception should be significantly minimized or removed by injecting the trigger area with a local anesthetic.

Time-honored treatment of the fibrositis syndrome consists mainly of local injections of an anesthetic agent into the trigger area once the trigger points and the referral zone have been identified. Similar benefit can also be obtained by spraying the tender area with ethyl-chloride or vasocoolant spray (Kraus, 1941). Deep sustained pressure manually exerted upon the trigger has been effective and has been termed acupressure. It is important to understand that the treatment must be aimed at the eradication of the trigger area and not specifically at the referred zone.

It is mandatory that precise systematic examination be performed on any patient with vague but painful disabling symptoms that suggest myofascial etiology. The physician must suspect the presence of triggers, and not dismiss them merely as having psychogenic origins simply because they do not follow classical neurological or orthopedic patterns. It also is mandatory that the precipitating and/or predisposing factors be discovered and eliminated. Diminished range of motion of involved joints should be treated with appropriate exercises directed toward correction of the postural components; occupational stresses should be evaluated and remedied. If depression or anxiety is deemed to be prominent, appropriate behavioral and psychological treatment obviously should be initiated.

Degenerative Arthritis: Symptomatic Osteoarthrosis

Degenerative arthritis is a common cause of organic, pathogenic pain. This medical condition has perhaps the highest morbidity of all human illnesses. It has been estimated that approximately 85 percent of all persons reaching the age of 70 have evidence of degenerative arthritis. In 1978 it was estimated that 180,000 persons in the United States were confined to bed or to a wheelchair as a direct result of osteoarthrosis or its manifestations.

Degenerative joint disease (DJD), otherwise termed osteoarthrosis or degenerative arthritis, is a disease of articulations, either peripheral or central, characterized by degeneration of cartilage with subsequent thickening of subchondral bone and gradual remodeling of bone and formation of marginal spurs.

Nociception occurs from tissue inflammation due to the evolution of faulty mechanics of the joint, loss of mobility of the injured joints, changes in the lubrication, and gradual development of joint instability. The nociceptive stimulation is related to tissue changes, the impairment of movement, the stresses imposed upon the articulations, and the specific sensitivity of the adjacent tissues involved by the degenerated joints.

Joint pathology has focused most attention upon the cartilage of the joint: its mechanism, structure, and metabolism. Joint lubrication also has received a great deal of attention. The study of symptomatic osteoarthrosis has focused on specific sites and their unique pathogenesis. The medical literature is replete with articles on lumbar spine degeneration, spinal stenosis, hip or knee arthritis, etc. Every entity currently enjoys a precise description of symptoms, a dissertation of probable causation factors or etiologies, an analysis of basis for symptoms, and a dialogue of treatment currently in vogue.

The human joint functions by virtue of its cartilage. Cartilage comprises essentially collagen and proteoglycans (PGs), with collagen forming half or more of its volume. The collagen fibrils are tightly interlaced and, besides acting as mechanical "springs," confine and compress the water-binding proteoglycan molecules. The chemistry of cartilage is intricate and undergoing constant revision. A full discussion is beyond the scope of this presentation and the reader is referred to the voluminous literature. The cartilage matrix binds up to 1000 times its weight in water and is essentially constrained by the collagen network.

By its imbibition of fluid and the imposed constraints, an intrinsic pressure can be created in the vicinity of 2.5 to 5 atmospheres.

Cartilage is compressible and elastic by virtue of the collagen network and its contained hydrodynamic fluid content. Joints function on the basis of compressibility and deformation. Lubrication is maintained by the intactness of cartilage and by compression (Cailliet, 1969).

Pathochemical changes in articular cartilage have a "natural" historical sequence regardless of the basic or primary causative factor. These primary factors can be listed simplistically as follows: (1) inflammatory disorders; (2) endocrine disorders; (3) metabolic disorders; (4) developmental disorders; and (5) physical factors, including (a) trauma, (b) disturbances in biomechanical balance, (c) altered subchondral circulation, (d) altered proprioception (neurogenic), and (e) altered properties of cartilage.

The nociceptive cycle begins with insult (injury) to the chondrocyte with release of destructive enzymes, particularly a protoeoglycanase. These enzymes affect the matrix and break it down (Barrett, 1975). As the matrix deteriorates, its water-binding capacity is decreased, with diminished capability to absorb its nutrients. The cartilage erodes, exposes the collagen fibers to wear, and the cushioning effect is lost. The exposed ends of the fibrils now can and do act as irritants. The lubricant is diminished (mucin, hyaluronidase, etc.) and the cycle progresses. As the cartilage erodes, fibrous tissue and then bone gradually replace the eroded area, producing the narrowed joint space, the irregular articulating surfaces, and the resultant nociceptive stimulation.

As the joint space narrows, the encircling capsule and ligaments slacken and the joints become progressively inflexible and unstable. The eroded surfaces tend to repair and do so with ebornation and osteophytosis. Hence further limitation and further deformation develop with increasing tissue irritation and impairment.

There are postulated biomechanical factors that are considered as causative in degenerative arthritis. In the aged (50–70), the hip, as an example, remodels itself constantly, thus changing the contour and its weight-bearing stresses. These stresses contribute to the ultimate degenerative arthritic changes of the cartilage. This process also is applicable to the knee and to its changes. Microscopic fractures have been noted in the trabecular bone immediately beneath the cartilage. This trabecular bone heals by calcification, which makes it then less resilient and more exposed to trauma. The circulation to the cartilage may also be impaired and thus becomes a further source of nociceptive stimulation.

Any trauma to any peripheral joint impairing normal joint movement can result in ultimate degenerative changes, mostly in weight-bearing joints, but not necessarily limited to them only.

Loads are not limited to weight-bearing joints but are related to forces applied by the muscles acting across the joints. Measurement of forces applied by calculating surface areas of contact with forces of muscular contraction would indicate that the joints of the upper extremity are under stress equal to that on the lower extremities.

The nature of joint lubrication remains unsettled between hydrodynamic principles (MacConaill, 1932), boundary phenomenon (Jones, 1934), and hydrostatic "weeping" (McCutchen, 1959). What is well accepted is that cartilage, upon pressure, exudes a viscous fluid that is a lubricant; the cartilage reabsorbs fluid by release of pressure (by imbibition). The lubricant fills the numerous crevices of the cartilage and decreases friction, wear, and tear. The constantly moving synovial fluid acts as a nutrient to the cartilage. Cartilage is an actively viable tissue and the chondrocytes are metabolically active and can repair themselves (Kettunen, 1958–59), usually by forming fibrocartilage (Shands, 1931).

Numerous studies designed to resolve the true causes of degenerative arthritis have so far failed to reach conclusive results (Sokoloff, 1969). Frictional forces exerted by mere rubbing are too weak to destroy cartilage (Radin et al., 1970). The synovial fluid of normal joints and of arthritic joints are equally effective lubricants, and so a change of synovial fluid per se is not the cause of joint degeneration (Linn & Radin, 1968), or at least does not initiate it. The main forces acting upon joints are longitudinal and therefore must be imposed by muscular contraction acting across the joint. Cartilage is extremely susceptible to stress (Mankin Lippiello, 1970) and the subchondral bone apparently bears much of the resilience of compressive forces. If the subchondral bone is stiffer, the cartilage is exposed to greater stress and degeneration.

In early degenerative arthritis, subchondral bone appears to be stiffer (Radin et al., 1970). Multiple microfractures of the subchondral bone heal by calcification and thus "stiffen" the subchondral bone (Radin et al., 1972). Continual exposure to stress probably allows ground substance of the cartilage to leak out, causing lysosomal activity to occur and thus initiating and furthering cartilage degeneration (Radin, 1972–73).

How joint degeneration causes painful perceptions is not fully understood (Steidler, 1959). There is effusion of the synovial fluid that contains sulfated mucopolysaccharides but the effect of this chemical is not known. Possible sources of nociceptive stimulation may be found in synovial reaction to cartilage changes with concomitant capsular changes; in irritation of nerve roots within the intervertebral foramina of the cervical, thoracic, and lumbar spine segments; in secondary muscle contractions to immobilize the ailing joints; and in other factors to be evaluated, indluding obesity, postural defects, and varus valgus.

Treatment modalities of splinting, exercising, intraarticular injections, anti-inflammatory medication, antimuscle spasm medicine, chemical denervation of joints by blocks, traction, etc., all should follow specific indication and specific procedures, which should be related to the specific nature of the predominant nociceptive focus.

"Chronic tension," of whatever etiology, causes sustained isometric muscle contraction of numerous joints of the body. This is particularly true of the cervical spine and disks and their facets. This tension undoubtedly generates sustained cartilaginous as well as intervertebral disk compression. The effect of continued tension of the periarticular muscles upon the subchondral bone is unknown, but chronically tense patients have been observed to have severe cervical disk degeneration. The disk degeneration noted in the cervical spine of patients months to years after a rear-end hyperflexion–hyperextension injury may well be explained by microtrauma, microfracture, and sustained tension.

The presence of "degenerative changes" in patients with chronic pain may not have etiological significance; this finding may simply be related, complicating, or even irrelevant. Merely finding radiological joint changes during the course of a medical investigation for chronic pain does not specifically identify the nociceptive source of the painful state, but merely presents an avenue to be wisely explored (Chapter 2).

REFERENCES

Bard, P. 1956. *Medical Physiology*. St. Louis: C.V. Mosby.

Barrett, A.J. 1975. In *Dynamics of Connective Tissue Macromolecules*, P.M.C. Burleigh and A.R. Poole (Eds.). Amsterdam: North-Holland, pp. 189–226.

Brendstrup, P., Jespersen, K., and Asboe-Hansen, G. 1957. Morphological and chemical connective tissue changes in fibrositic muscles. *Ann. Rheumat. Dis.* 16: 438–440.

Cailliet, R. 1969. Mechanics of joints. In *Arthritis in Physical Medicine*, E. Licht and S. Licht (Eds.). Baltimore: Waverly Press.

Cailliet, R. 1977. *Soft Tissue Pain and Disability*. Philadelphia: F.A. Davis.

Cooper, A.L. 1961. Trigger-point injection: Its place in physical medicine. *Arch. Phys. Med. Rehab.* 42: 704–709.

Jones, E.S. 1934. Joint lubrication. *Lancet* 1:1426–1427.

Kettunen, K.O. 1958–1959. Cartilaginous metaplasia of connective tissue in clinical skin arthroplasty. *Acta Orthopaed. Scand.* 28: 190–197.

Kraft, G.H., Johnson, E.W., and LaBan, M.M. 1968. The fibrositis syndrome. *Arch. Phys. Med. Rehab.* 49: 155–162.

Kraus, H. 1941. The use of surface anesthesia in the treatment of painful motion. *JAMA* 116: 2582–2583.

Linn, F.C., and Radin, E.L. 1968. Lubrication of animal joints. III. The effect of certain chemical alterations of the cartilage and lubricant. *Arthrit. Rheumat.* 11: 674–682.

MacConaill, M.A. 1932. The function of intra-articular fibro-cartilages, with special reference to the knee and inferior radio-ulnar joints. *J. Anat.* 66: 210–227.

Mankin, H.J., and Lippiello, L. 1970. Biochemical and metabolic abnormalities in articular cartilage from osteo-arthritic human hips. *J. Bone J. Surg.* 52A: 424–434.

McCutchen, C.W. 1959. Mechanism of animal joints: Spongehydrostatic and weeping bearings. *Nature* 184: 1284–1285.

Michele, A.A., Davies, J.J., Krueger, F.J., and Lichtor, J.M. 1950. Scapulocostal syndrome (Fatigue-Postural Paradox). *N.Y. State J. Med.* 50: 1353–1356.

Moldofsky, H., Scarisbrick, P., England, R., and Smythe, H. 1975. Musculoskeletal symptoms and non-REM sleep disturbances in patients with "fibrositis syndrome" and healthy subjects. *Psychosomat. Med.* 37: 341–351.

Radin, E.L. 1972–1973. The physiology and degeneration of joints. *Sem. Arthrit. Rheumat.* 2: 245–257.

Radin, E.L., Paul, I.L., and Pollock, D. 1970. Animal joint behaviour under excessive loading. *Nature* 226: 554–555.

Radin, E.L., Paul, I.L., and Tolkoff, M.J. 1970. Subchondral bone changes in patients with early degenerative joint disease. *Arthrit. Rheumat.* 13: 400–405.

Radin, E.L., Pugh, J.W., Steinberg, R.S., et al. 1972. Trabecular micro-fracture in response to stress. *Proceedings of the XII SICOT Congress.*

Shands, A.R. 1931. The regeneration of hyaline cartilage in joints: An experimental study. *Arch. Surg.* 22: 137–178.

Smythe, H.A., and Moldofsky, H. 1977–1978 series. Two contributions to understanding of the fibrositis syndrome. *Bull. Rheumat. Dis.* 1: 928–931.

Sokoloff, L. 1969. *The Biology of Degenerative Joint Disease.* Chicago: University of Chicago Press.

Sola, A.E., and Kuitert, J.H. 1955. Myofascial trigger point pain in the neck and shoulder girdle: Report of 100 cases treated by injection of normal saline. *Northwest Med.* 54: 980–984.

Steidler, A. 1959. *Lectures on the Interpretation of Pain in Orthopedic Practice.* Springfield, Ill.: Charles C. Thomas, pp 61–64.

Travell, J., and Rinzler, S.H. 1952. The myofascial genesis of pain. *Postgrad. Med.* 11: 425–434.

Webster's New Twentieth Century Dictionary 1978 (unabridged, second edition). Englewood Cliffs, N.J.: Collins World Publishing.

Weinberger, L.M. 1977. Traumatic fibromyositis: A critical review of an enigmatic concept. *West. J. Med.* 127: 99–103.

8

Causalgia and the Deafferentiation Syndromes

BENJAMIN L. CRUE, JR.

Major causalgia *is usually caused by an open wound involving a mixed peripheral nerve. Pain develops that typically demonstrates two characteristics: (1) it is made worse by light touch, and (2) there is an element of constant pain, often burning in character.* Minor causalgia *is a poorly defined group of syndromes, and usually indicates psychopathology, often premorbid and not just reactive to the pain. The treatment for major causalgia is* prompt *sympathetic nerve block and/or surgical sympathectomy. The treatment for minor causalgia is* not *surgical, but psychotherapy, often best administered within a group setting, and occasionally needing a multidisciplinary pain team approach, especially for cases with reflex sympathetic dystrophy.* Deafferentiation *means loss of peripheral afferent input, believed to lead under many circumstances to central hyperirritability or excitatory states.*

DEFINITIONS

In the United States, the term causalgia dates back at least to the writings of Weir Mitchell (Walter, 1970) and his description of the syndrome following war wounds during the American Civil War. The Greek derivation of the word *causalgia* comes from "heat" plus "pain"; and causalgia is defined as a neuralgia characterized by intense local sensation as of a burning pain. *Algia* is defined merely as a suffix indicating a relation to pain. *Neuralgia*, "nerve" plus "pain," is defined as pain in a nerve, or in nerves, or radiating along the course of the nerve (implied also is the concept of "unknown cause").

There are many specific neuralgias, many known by the proper name of the physician generally credited with first describing the particular clinical syndrome, such as Fothergill's neuralgia (of the trigeminal nerve), Hunt's neuralgia (geniculate ganglion neuralgia, usually postherpetic), Morton's neuralgia (between the third and fourth toe), or Sluder's neuralgia (of the sphenopalatine gaglion, giving the so-called "shawl" neuralgia). Or the neuralgia may be entirely described by giving the general anatomical location in which the pain is felt, such as cardiac neuralgia (for angina pectoris), facial neuralgia (for pain in the face), intercostal neuralgia (for pain in the distribution of the intercostal nerves over the thorax), or occipital neuralgia (for pain in the back of the head).

CENTRAL MECHANISM

The present author, in Chapter 3 on the neurophysiology of pain, has presented his bias as a "centralist" when it comes to chronic pain syndromes. He must admit in this chapter that he has an even stronger prejudice regarding his conceptualization of mechanism in *-algia:* —Algia is a pain generated *centrally* that is *referred peripherally* into the distribution of a peripheral or cranial nerve. Although the patient may subjectively feel as if the pain were originating in the anatomical region of the peripheral or cranial nerve where the pain is felt; and while, in many instances, there may well have been an original etiological organic peripheral lesion (usually within that distribution) that apparently started the neuralgia syndrome (which of necessity reinforces the patient's and the physician's belief in the pain mechanism as having something to do with the peripheral area where both the pain is felt and the original causative tissue trauma on many occasions has occurred and there is now "scar"), it remains this author's opinion that the neurophysiological mechanism underlying neuralgic pain is entirely central (Livingston, 1944).

Furthermore, it is most likely that repetitive firing in low-level neuronal aggregates can also be considered to be a form of sensory epilepsy, as in trigeminal neuralgia (Crue et al., 1964). The same phenomena are likely to be involved in various other painful syndromes with peripheral neuralgic jabbing pains, including causalgia with its peripheral visceral afferent, its central autonomic, and its reflex efferent or sensory antidromic components. It is assumed that the neuronal network involved in the lancinating pains of neuralgia and in causalgia are probably closer to the primary afferent endings, with either a different or an additive more central and cephalad sensory network involved in the more prolonged constant pains usually seen in the chronic intractable benign pain syndrome patient.

-ALGIA, -ITIS, AND -OPATHY

It is important that the reader also realize the specific differences between "-algia," "-itis," and "-opathy" as related to pain syndromes (Wartenberg,

1958). *Neuritis* results from an inflammation in the nerve (whether it is due to bacterial infection, viral infection, the inflammation that accompanies diabetic "neuropathy," or even compression entrapment syndromes), and is apparently a cause of pain only in acute, subacute, or recurrent acute pain syndromes; -itis is *not* usually a peripheral causative agent for any continued nociceptive input in chronic pain syndromes. *Neuropathy* refers to pathology or damage within the nerve, in the absence of inflammation (that is, no accompanying "neuritis"). Neuropathy, such as that seen in many slowly degenerative diseases, usually is not painful. *Neuralgia* may start with a neuropathy or a neuritis, and the pain syndrome becomes established only when the central mechanism takes over. The pain of neuralgia signifies an underlying central mechanism that is referring the pain peripherally.

Since the central mechanism is usually established in an anatomical location spatially involving the area of nociceptive input from the site of the etiological injury, it is highly likely that the neuralgic pain will be referred back to the area of the original peripheral pathology. This is not always so, as in ulnar pain in the left arm in response to damage of the myocardium, where there is a central overlap involving the area of input from both peripheral sensory distributions entering at the T1 level. (However, there is more to the central cervical "pain pool" than a single level, as myocardial damage also often causes pain referred all the way up to and into the trigeminal area, usually in the mandibular division of V.) But this classical example, while showing central overlap in acute pain, is very rarely considered in relation to chronic neuralgic syndromes.

One of the most common distant neuralgic referred pain syndromes is seen in occipital neuralgia. Here pain is felt in the distribution of the greater occipital nerve, but it is probably referred there from a central mechanism that, in most instances, is established in response to damage and acute nociceptive input in the mid or lower cervical region, which is subject to the most trauma. In the opinion of this author, greater occipital neuralgia is seldom if ever due to entrapment of the C2 posterior primary division itself, but is usually a referred pain from central mechanisms overlapping with the midcervical peripheral input dermatones (Crue et al., 1964). (This C2 posterior primary division centrally overlaps most often with the ophthalmic division of V.)

Diabetic neuropathy is usually originally painful because of associated inflammation but there may well be other peripheral factors, such as demyelinization with "cross-talk" at the site of the peripheral etiological causative lesion in the usually "mixed" nerve. However, the subsequent constant chronic pain, as well as the lancinating jabs of pain that are seen so often (and are so hard to treat in diabetics), is almost always a neuralgia reflecting a central mechanism.

Post-herpetic neuralgia starts with a viral neuritis, and progresses to a neuropathy; but the pain is quite correctly labeled (unlike diabetic neuropathy) as a neuralgia because the central mechanism continues to refer the pain back along the damaged nerve long after all inflammation has subsided. There is still considerable room for doubt, however, as to just how the central mechanism is established in post-herpetic neuralgia. A known inflammation due to the herpes virus not only causes damage at the site of the "shingles" at the cutaneous endings of the peripheral nerve, but also can cause obvious damage in the dorsal ganglion, in the dorsal root, and even into the spinal cord itself. In post-herpetic neuralgia, therefore, there well may be a central pathological lesion as well as a central physiological hyperactivity neuronal state from deafferentiation. In most cases of neuralgia, the central hypersensitivity state can be established on a neurophysiological basis alone, after pathological damage in the periphery resulting in interruption of or altered patterns of afferent inputs (deafferentiation hypersensitivity). This mechanism is likely involved in causalgic syndromes following a gunshot wound to the median nerve in the wrist in a patient with a presumed normal central nervous system. The existence of "command neurones" in the dorsal horn subserving pain has been discussed elsewhere (Crue & Carregal, 1975).

The reason for discussing possible central mechanisms in these neuralgic and/or deafferentiation states is that such an understanding may play a key role in treatment. For example, it is no wonder that iatrogenic destruction of the peripheral apparatus in such a central pain state may serve no useful purpose for any significant length of time, in any significant percentage of patients, with pain from postherpetic neuralgia. Neither destruction of the skin under the site of the healed lesions nor nerve block of the involved peripheral nerve itself, nor even dorsal root rhizotomy, has proved over the years to be sufficiently efficacious to justify use in the human with post-herpetic neuralgia. It can be stated most forcefully that ablative surgery is contraindicated in post-herpetic neuralgia.

Conversely, if the underlying neurophysiological mechanism is central, then perhaps it makes more empirical sense, both clinically and neurophysiologically, to direct treatment toward the central nervous system site of the neuralgic syndromes.

IMPORTANCE OF MEMORY

The problem of taxonomy related specifically to these deafferentiation pain syndromes is also difficult. Many are rare syndromes. Others are much more common, but the numerous reported treatments and varying reported results have led to much confusion in the treatment of such hypersensitivity pain states.

Ramzy and Wallerstein (1958) presented a psychoanalytical schematization of pain (Fig. 8-1) that remains useful to this day. We would take their classification of "neurotic bodily pain" ("no discernible stimulus to the body,

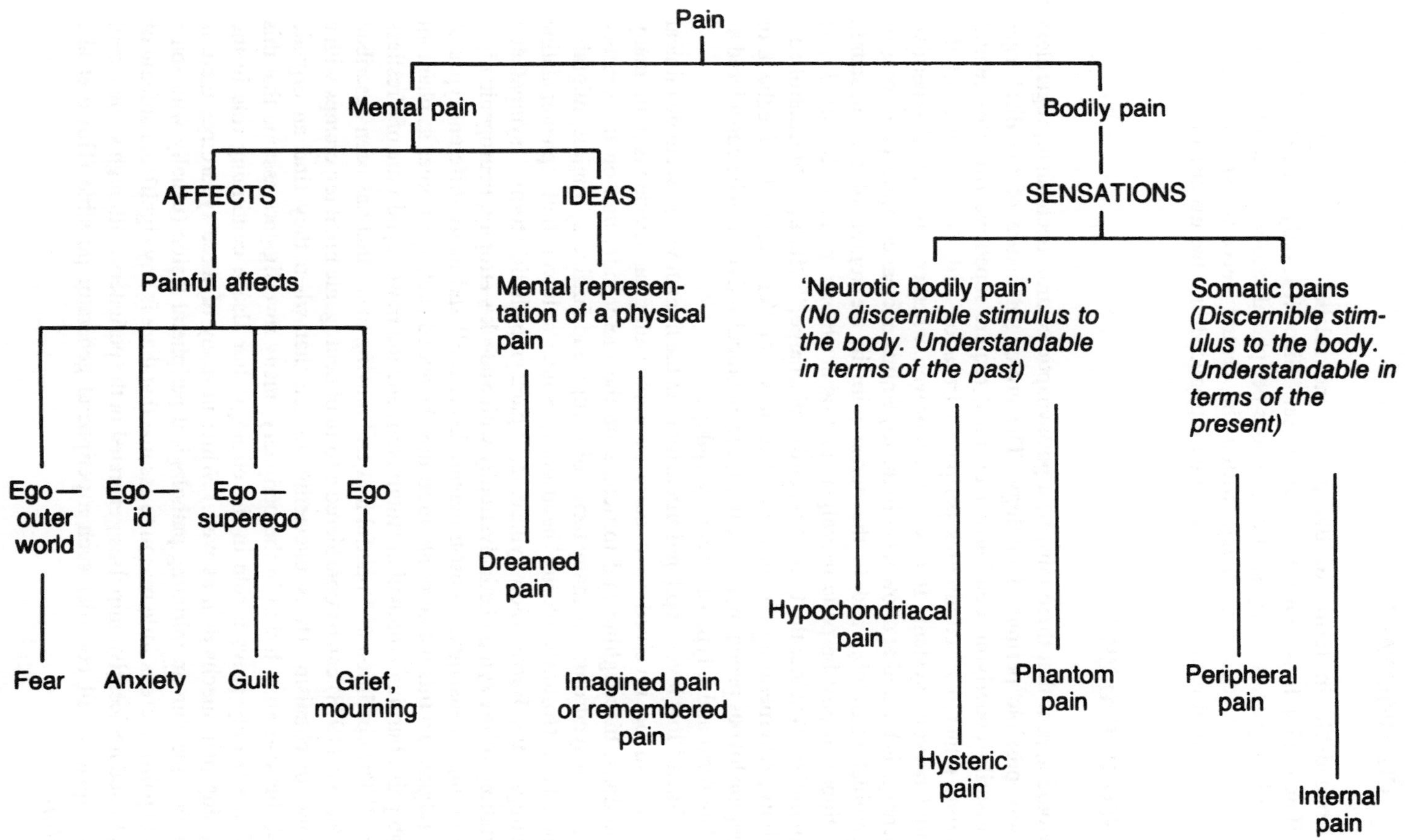

FIG. 8-1. Psychoanalytic schematization of pain (From Ramzy & Wallerstein, 1958)

understandable in terms of the past") and relabel it as "-algia and the deafferentiation hypersensitivity pain states." Since it is only understandable in terms of the past, it is implied that previous peripheral sensory input information has somehow caused a change within the central nervous system, and the phenomenon of *memory* now has to be introduced into the discussion.

SENSORY EPILEPSY

It would appear that there must be a postsynaptic central mechanism, regardless of any possible peripheral etiology. The prolonged nature of the discharges necessarily underlying continued pain must require repetitive firing of central neurons rather than continuous peripheral irritation with bombardment of the central nervous system. It is yet to be proven whether this central repetitive discharge is located at a low level in the trigeminal nuclear complex in the case of trigeminal neuralgia, and in the dorsal horn in the region of the substantia gelatinosa in post-herpetic neuralgias and other chronic pains of the trunk and extremities. Whether the terms "repetitive discharge," "flare," "uncontrolled" activity, reverberating circuit pain, "memory" or "engrammed," feedback or other analogous pseudonyms are used, this neuronal activity can be considered as epileptiform and a type of "sensory epilepsy."

Such "low level" epileptiform activity in the human would seem on clinical grounds to be involved as a basic neurophysiological mechanism in many conditions; hiccoughing and torticollis on the motor side; and on the sensory side, such syndromes as many forms of vertigo and dizziness, tinnitus, migraine headaches, Horton's cluster headaches, Sluder's lower half sphenopalatine neuralgia, the Barre–Liou syndrome, "parasympathetic storm," sympathetic irritation, reflex sympathetic dystrophy with Sudeck's atrophy, neurogenic night leg cramps, causalgia, "post-traumatic headache" and many different types of neuralgias. To this list certainly must now be added such syndromes as phantom limb pain, burning amputation stump pain, and the newer syndrome of "restless legs." The condition of "painful legs and moving toes" that has been described by Nathan (1978) can be considered a form of neurogenic night leg cramps with a central mechanism. (It is interesting to see that when they find an organic probable-causative lesion in the periphery, many investigators assume that this lesion not only plays a role in the etiology, but also a continuing role in the ongoing pain mechanism as well.) While in many of these syndromes there is without question an initiating pathological peripheral lesion (usually with some acute pain), there is little reason to assume that there is any significant amount of continued nociceptive impulses generated in the periphery, although some recent investigators still consider such a peripheral generator possible (Howe et al., 1978).

TWO TYPICAL KINDS OF PAIN IN NEURALGIA AND CAUSALGIA

In these neuralgic pain syndromes, there generally appear to be two different kinds of subjective pain. It is believed that in both there is an underlying central mechanism referring the pain back to the periphery.

The first type is the obvious lancinating jabbing pains of intermittent neuralgia. These jabs are probably due to a more peripheral sensory neuronal network, at a very low level near the primary afferent endings; they are helped in most instances by treatment with anticonvulsants, such as Dilantin and Tegretol.

The second type is a constant pain, usually referred very superficially to the dermis, generally in the area where the original pathology may have been. For example, pain is usually felt in (and often triggered from touch in) the same intercostal area where the scars of the shingles are most prominent. Constant burning superficial pain is often felt in the amputation stump in some patients, with or without painful stump neuromas, or in phantom limb pain. These more constant chronic pain syndromes, in a very high percentage, are apt to have a burning quality; however, occasionally there may be no burning but rather a feeling of cold. We have no idea as to the differences in the abnormal central readout that perceives "hot" in most, but "cold" in a few, patients (Crue et al., 1979). The important thing from the treatment standpoint is that this more constant type of pain is *not* helped by anticonvulsant medications. Instead it appears to respond, at least partially, in many cases, to antidepressant medication, either amitriptyline or doxepin. However, such treatment for the constant pain by the use of antidepressants does not have as high a clinical success rate for total pain suppression as the anticonvulsants do for neuralgic jabs.

Why do psychotropic drugs help chronic syndromes with constant pain? Is it because there are higher central descending mechanisms (perhaps in the limbic system) which potentiate a lower central repetitively firing epileptiform mechanism? Are these mechanisms the same as those associated with psychiatric states such as anxiety, guilt, or grief over loss? Or is there a true neuropharmacological effect at a lower level? Is it perhaps related to the obviously multifaceted newly discovered complex endorphin and enkephalin systems, with their connections with the hypothalamic axis?

MAJOR CAUSALGIA

In our experience acute major causalgia is usually due to known severe organic damage, usually with a penetrating wound, to a mixed (sensory and motor) peripheral nerve. However, there is generally more to primary causalgia than just pain with a burning quality referred to the distribution of the injured nerve. The proper diagnosis of major causalgia requires two qualities: (1) it should be made much worse by a *light touch* on the skin, usually in the involved area; and (2) there should be an element of chronic *constant pain* that is often accompanied by evidence of sympathetic dysfunction (such as profuse sweating, or color changes in the affected extremity), and usually (but not necessarily) an element of *burning or heat*. However, there are true causalgic syndromes with no burning quality or even with feelings of cold.

The time sequence in the development of major causalgia is of interest. If the pain were attributable entirely to a gradual establishment of a central deafferentiation hyperactivity state, from loss of peripheral afferents, one would expect that it would occur slowly; however there may be immediate onset. Furthermore one would expect that it would be seen after lesions of purely sensory nerves, but the lesions usually occur in mixed sensory and motor nerves. In many instances of causalgia, therefore, there is an initial etiological peripheral element of cross-talk at the site of the mixed nerve injury. This process has been well described by Granit (1955), and has even been suggested hypothetically by Gardner as playing a possible role in trigeminal neuralgia (although there are no known motor efferent fibers in the peripheral trigeminal system).

The peripheral mechanisms of the cross-talk phenomenon from peripheral injury are still entirely in the realm of conjecture; however, in major causalgia the central hyperactivity state is established and clinically manifested quickly. It has long been known that surgical intervention or sympathetic nerve blocks must be performed early and properly to have any significant effect on the causalgic syndrome.

Treatment

The standard treatment for acute severe major causalgia is *prompt* sympathetic nerve block for the involved extremity. If pain recurs after such a sympathetic block, or at most after a short series of blocks, then prompt surgical sympathectomy should usually be carried out. The longer the delay in instituting such appropriate therapy, the poorer are the results.

By definition, the autonomic nervous system, both sympathetic and parasympathetic, is entirely motor (Pick, 1970). Visceral afferents from the vessels, the muscles, and the visceral organs transverse the autonomic chain, although their cell bodies lie within the dorsal root ganglion. It still is not clear if the changes in painful intensity are brought about by actual block of the sympathetic motor efferents, or by interruption of the visceral afferents from the painful area as they cross the sympathetic ganglia. The well established value of sympathectomy in providing long-term relief of causalgic pain may be due to the same mechanism. While this hypothesis is still unproven it is possible that a more complete deafferentiation by interruption of the appropriate afferents to partially deafferentiated central neuronal networks may alter the normal repetitive firing and thus provide clinical improvement.

Why is it that deafferentiation may be at the same time a cause of central pain states and a treatment modality? This question has been addressed in the experimental animal laboratory concerning mechanisms of trigeminal neuralgia and not of causalgia. (However, both syndromes share likely neurological central mechanisms). It is known that experimental implantation of aluminum gel in the trigeminal spinal nucleus (Black, 1970) using a techinque similar to Kennard (1953) in the spinal cord, can produce in the cat both epileptiform discharges from the trigeminal nucleus and a hypersensitive state in the face, as evidenced by its not allowing its whiskers or hair to be touched. A trigeminal rhizotomy will then cure the "pain syndrome" in the animal. On the other hand, merely doing a trigeminal rhizotomy (and causing deafferentiation of the trigeminal nucleus) in a normal cat can produce apparently *non painful* epileptiform activity, which also can be recorded by electrodes within the trigeminal nucleus of the cat's brain stem. There is probably a different neuronal network involved under these two different conditions. However, it is ironic that rhizotomy can cause laboratory epileptiform activity by deafferentiation hypersensitivity, when it is a standard clinical treatment for trigeminal neuralgia. The demonstration that human trigeminal evoked potentials recorded from the spinal trigeminal nucleus appear more epileptiform in a tic patient than in a cancer pain patient during trigeminal stereotactic tractotomy is still tenuous and must be duplicated by others (Crue et al., 1975).

With major causalgia, it appears that input over the visceral afferents is specifically related to the burning pain, with its obvious resultant sympathetic dysfunction indicating an altered efferent output to the small blood vessels of the involved extremity. While properly done sympathetic nerve blocks and sympathectomy are almost universally successful in relieving the painful state of early major causalgia, it is of clinical interest that many patients are relieved by beta-adrenergic blockers such as propranolol.

MINOR CAUSALGIA

Minor causalgia is a poorly defined pain syndrome, which also is sometimes called secondary causalgia, second-order causalgia, closed-injury causalgia, causalgia without known damage to a peripheral nerve, etc. Clinically, there are a large number of patients with a "wastebasket" full of chronic pain problems with some causalgic symptoms, but with no history of severe injury (especially no open wound of mixed peripheral nerve), no sign of cutaneous hypersensitivity to light touch, and no burning feelings. Evidence of sympathetic dysfunction may also be absent, or develop at a later stage of the painful process.

Most of the very late sequelae of efferent reflex dystrophy, such as Sudeck's atrophy and severe osteoporosis, contracture of the joints, and peripheral edema, are also common signs of disuse. These symptoms have *not* been seen in patients with primary causalgia that had not been promptly or properly treated. Instead they were seen in patients with a secondary or minor type of causalgia, for which their physician did not believe that block or sympathectomy was indicated. These patients developed over a long period of time a full-blown Sudeck's component of the total pain syndrome.

Treatment

At the present time, the author is not aware of any good medical or surgical treatment for these chronic cases. Propranolol does not help, and sympathectomy usually does not help very much. It has become more and more obvious over the years that patients with this type of minor causalgia, which develops into a more severe chronic pain syndrome, almost always have underlying severe psychopathology. This psychopathology is usually not entirely reactive, but rather there is a life history of chaos, the existence of secondary gain (such as unsettled litigation or Workers' Compensation), or a premorbid personality structure predisposed to the development of a pain of chronic intractable benign pain syndromes (as discussed in Chapter 3 on neurophysiology). Treatment in this group is extremely difficult indeed. Our few successes have been attained by the use of group psychotherapy, and by the utilization of the entire multidisciplinary pain team. At present there is no known surgical or medical treatment per se for this type of severe chronic pain syndrome, with sympathetic system elements (Frazier, 1966), and poor patient coping.

REFERENCES

Black, R. 1970. Trigeminal pain. In *Pain and Suffering: Selected Aspects,* B.L. Crue (Ed.). Charles C. Thomas Springfield, Ill.

Crue, B.L., Carregal, E.J.A., and Todd, E.M. 1964. Neuralgia—Discussion of central mechanisms. *Bull. L.A. Neurol. Soc. 29:107.*

Crue, B.L., Todd, E.M., and Carregal, E.J.A. 1970. Observations on the present status of the compression procedure in trigeminal neuralgia. In *Pain and Suffering: Selected Aspects,* B.L. Crue (Ed.). Springfield, Ill.: Charles C. Thomas.

Crue, B.L., and Carregal, E.J.A. 1975. Pain begins in the dorsal horn—With a suggested classification of the primary senses. In *Pain: Research and Treatment,* B.L. Crue (Ed.). New York: Academic Press.

Crue, B.L., Carregal, E.J.A., and Felsoory, A. 1975. Percutaneous stereotactic radiofrequency trigeminal tractotomy with neurophysiological recordings. In *Pain: Research and Treatment,* B.L. Crue (Ed.). New York: Academic Press.

Crue, B.L., Felsoory, A., and Pinsky, J.J. 1979. Temperature triggered contralateral "neuralgic" pain following "Nashold procedure" for phantom pain. *Chronic Pain: Further Observations From City of Hope National Medical Center,* (B.L. Crue (Ed.). New York: Spectrum.

Frazier, S.H. 1966. Psychiatric aspects of causalgia, the phantom limb, and phantom pain. *Dis. Nerv. Sys.* 27:442.

Granit, R. 1955. *Receptors and Sensory Perception.* New Haven: Yale University Press.

Howe, J.F., Loeser, J.D., and Calvin, W.H., 1978. Mechanosensitivity of dorsal root ganglia and chronically injured axons. A physiological basis for the radicular pain of nerve root compression. Second World Congress on Pain, Montreal, Canada, August 27–September 1.

Kennard, M.A. 1953. Sensitization of the spinal cord of the cat to pain-inducing stimuli. *J. Neurosurg.* 10:169.

Livingston, W.K. 1944. *Pain Mechanisms, A Physiologic Interpretation of Causalgia and Its Related States.* New York: Macmillan.

Nathan, P.W. 1978. Painful legs and moving toes: Evidence on the site of the lesion. *J. Neurol. Neurosurg. Psychiatr.* 41:934.

Pick, J. 1970. *The Autonomic Nervous System.* Philadelphia: J.B. Lippincott.

Ramzy, I., and Wallerstein, R.S. 1958. Pain, fear and anxiety. A study in their inter-relationships. *Psychoanal. Study Child.* 13:147.

Walter, R.D. 1970. *S. Weir Mitchell, M.D., Neurologist. A Medical Biography.* Springfield, Ill.: Charles C. Thomas.

Wartenberg, R. 1958. *Neuritis, Sensory Neuritis, and Neuralgia.* New York: Oxford University Press.

9

Psychological Assessment of Chronic Pain

STEPHEN J. JOHNSON

The variety and complexity of etiological factors that give rise to a chronic pain condition frequently make assessment inexact. Psychological theories and procedures that improve the quality of assessment are discussed in this chapter. In addition, information is provided on integrating assessment data. The final section covers future directions in the psychological assessment of chronic pain.

A great deal of ambiguity exists in the assessment of chronic pain conditions. The complexity and variety of etiological factors that give rise to a chronic pain condition frequently make diagnosis inexact. Melzack (1973) has observed that pain exists within the unique multidimensional frame of reference of the individual and, as such, is difficult to define. Wolff (1978) observes that ". . . in discussing pain measurement, the obvious fact must be emphasized that it is not easy to measure something if one is not sure what one is actually measuring."

In response to these ambiguities, behaviorists have attempted to quantify environmental factors and patient responses whenever possible. This quantification allows the use of a "data base" in place of solely "clinical judgment." The best controlled study to date of clinical judgment with chronic pain patients reveals its inadequacy (Fordyce et al., 1978). One hundred consecutive patients were referred to a university hospital pain clinic for evaluation of their problems. The patients were classified along an "organic—nonorganic" continuum based on ratings derived from a full set of medical diagnostic information that each patient had accrued. A mean interjudge correlation of 0.568 for diagnostic decisions was obtained, indicating only modestly better-than-chance agreement among the judges. Results such as this speak to the need to minimize clinical judgment when assessing pain patients and the need to objectify the assessment process as much as possible.

PSYCHOGENIC PAIN: A DYSFUNCTIONAL CONCEPT

The search for objective data when assessing the psychological factors in a chronic pain condition has often been hampered by the unfortunate dichotomy of "real" pain versus "psychogenic" pain. The diagnostic label of psychogenic pain implies that the etiology of the patient's pain problem is in the mind; that is, the patient does not have organic pain. Conversely patients who have demonstrable organic pathology that matches the amount of pain or illness behavior they emit may be viewed as having real pain and being honest and nonmanipulative. Patients with the label of psychogenic pain, however, often are viewed as "crocks" and as manipulative. One of the frequent goals for such patients is to have health care professionals believe them. Thus they may view surgery as exactly what is needed both to alleviate their pain problem and to give authenticity to their situation.

Besides leading the patient into treatment for the wrong reasons, the diagnosis of psychogenic pain provides little useful information in the way of therapeutic intervention. The psychodynamic issues that give rise to a psychogenic pain problem are difficult to assess and concrete suggestions for treatment frequently are not available.

Another problem with the diagnosis of psychogenic pain is that it frequently is formulated on the basis of no discernible organic pathology. Thus a positive diagnosis of one clinical condition is made on the basis of a lack of evidence of another clinical condition. One is reminded of the situation in which Alice told the king: "I see nobody on the road." The king's reply was, of course: "I only wish I had such eyes . . . to be able to see nobody, and at that distance too!" If a diagnosis suggesting a significant psychological component in a patient's pain problem is proposed, then that diagnosis should be established on the basis of positive psychological test and interview data, not on the lack of organic pathology.

The patient with a significant learned psychological component in a pain problem must be distinguished from the patient who attempts deliberately to deceive health care professionals in order to attain certain goals. Such a goal might be obtaining disability income contingent on pain behavior. Inaccurate diagnosis of deception can perpetuate a situation in which both the patient and insurance carrier lose. Patients lose because they do not understand the price that continued malingering extracts in decreased quality of life. Validity scales on psychological tests such as the Minnesota Multiphasic Personality Inventory are frequently useful in detecting this type of patient.

As discussed in other chapters throughout this book, the traditional disease model has utility for the understanding of acute pain problems. However, if pain behaviors persist long after an injury has been sustained, the disease model approach to assessing the patient may not be applicable, and a behavioral model approach should be considered.

Pain behavior can be classified, as indicated in Chapter 5, as "operant" (determined by its consequences) or "respondent" (a situation in which physical or environmental events that occur prior to the pain experience are critical). The fact that a problematic pain condition is primarily respondent in etiology does not necessarily mean that a learned maladaptive component is absent. Conditioned respondent pain often occurs through classical conditioning procedures and can be as debilitating as an operant pain problem.

DOLORIC, STOIC AND ASSIMILATED PAIN PATIENTS

Steger et al. (1980) have developed a conceptual framework that relabels operant pain patients as "doloric," but subdivides respondent pain into two distinct clinical conditions, stoic and assimilated. The utility of this extension of the operant–respondent classification is that it has greater treatment implications than the previous model.

Doloric Pain Patients

The doloric patient shows operant pain behavior. An example of this condition would be the case of a man with peripheral neuropathy whose pain behavior increased markedly when his wife, who had multiple sclerosis, was no longer able to care for herself. A behavioral analysis revealed that the patient's pain behavior was highest during the weekends when the daughter was visiting. The daughter would perform nursing care for the mother only if the father's pain was of such intensity that he was unable to perform the care. Thus, a doloric condition appeared to have developed because of the daughter's contingent performance of a task that the patient found unpleasant.

This case illustrates the point that a nonproblematic pain condition can form the basis for a totally different type of clinical pain condition. An important observation is that the patient's "suffering" actually increased when it became contingent upon the daughter's weekend visits. This observation suggests a potentially positive prognosis as alternative adaptive behaviors can be learned in the place of the learned maladaptive ones.

With doloric pain, behavior modification programs such as those discussed in Chapters 13 and 14 are useful in promoting health behaviors. The use of modalities such as surgery, medication, nerve blocks, or transcutaneous electrical stimulation are likely to be ineffective in the absence of psychological intervention.

Stoic Pain Patients

Stoic patients are seen by Steger et al. (1980) as being individuals who exhibit little overt pain behavior, tend to underutilize health care services and medication, and, in so far as possible, deny that they have a pain problem. These individuals often have conditioned respondent pain. They are active and refuse to modify their life-style in response to pain. Unlike the doloric patients, stoic patients do not show pain behavior in response to environmental rewards.

Stoic patients tend to be productive and energetic people who seem to be always in motion. For them the reinforcing aspect of being active is more powerful than the punishing aspect of the pain itself. Because personal achievement and productivity are very strongly reinforced in our society, many of these patients do not modulate their activity levels, and thus experience an exacerbation of their pain problems. This exacerbation may result from an energy drain associated with a high arousal or stress state. Also, these patients' organic pathology may worsen as a result of low compliance with therapeutic recommendations.

An example of a stoic patient would be a man who was greatly distressed by having lost six weeks of work for a laminectomy and was determined to catch up on his work. Thus he worked 10 to 12 hours per day and did not take breaks, even though he was experiencing severe pain. His condition continued to deteriorate until it was only with great effort that he was able to perform the work that was assigned to him, although he continued to state categorically that he was able to handle the demands of his employment. He entered a chronic pain program at the insistence of his employer and family physician, having worked up to the day before admission to the program.

Careful instruction and education about the nature of their condition and proper use of medication and activities are important in the treatment of stoic patients. These patients may respond well to modalities such as transcutaneous nerve stimulation, biofeedback, and nerve blocks, as well as to stress-management techniques to reduce arousal. Counseling to help them accept limitations may be especially helpful. On the other hand, ill-advised surgery, drastic curtailing of activities, or habit-forming medication may move stoic patients to a doloric state.

Assimilated Pain Patients

Assimilated pain patients are individuals who have managed to make the required adjustments in their life-style in order to remain as active as possible despite their pain problem. These patients typically use low amounts of medication, intelligently utilize health care services, and are able to manage activity levels effectively. One of the frequent treatment goals of therapy with stoic and doloric patients is to teach them the self-management skills that assimilated pain patients possess. Problems can occur if assimilated patients are misdiagnosed and inappropriately treated because of a desire on the part of health-care providers to "do something" for the chronic pain problem. The primary treatment goal with assimilated pain patients is maintenance of an assimilated pain state through education.

PSYCHOLOGICAL ASSESSMENT OF CHRONIC PAIN

Results from a psychological assessment of chronic pain need to be paired with medical findings to obtain a comprehensive evaluation. This section presents a survey of some aspects of psychological assessment that are in general usage.

History of Pain Problem

A thorough and detailed history of the patient's pain problem is essential as a base from which to evaluate and understand other information. This history should delineate what important environmental events occur prior to or after significant changes in the patient's pain problems and how the patient and family respond to these events and changes. The behavioral analysis described in the following usually is initiated using historical information.

Behavioral Analysis of Chronic Pain

The primary goal of a behavioral analysis of chronic pain is to determine the controlling and contributing factors in a person's pain behavior. It examines individual samples of behavior such as the specific responses made by family members when a patient demonstrates certain types of pain behavior. Thus, behavior is broken down into its individual components and the environmental factors controlling each component are analyzed separately. A behavioral analysis usually is accomplished through interviews with the patient and spouse. These interviews are usually done separately so that neither person feels constricted in providing information. Other family members and/or friends frequently prove to be good sources of information.

An assessment of behavior such as time spent in activities, medication taken, and verbal pain complaints can be objectified by directly observing the patient's behavior, or can be based on the patient's self-reports and/or on the family's reports. While direct observation may yield more accurate information, behavior can be influenced by the mere fact that it is being observed. It may be practical to rely heavily on the patient's self-reports, but to check them against reports from the family and through observations of the patient's behavior during treatment. The reader is referred to Fordyce (1976) for an elaboration of the details of this evaluation.

Assessment Issues with Doloric Pain

There are four main environmental factors that may contribute to the development of doloric pain: (1) positive reinforcement of pain behavior, (2) removal of an aversive state as a consequence of pain behavior, (3) low-frequency reinforcement of "well" behavior, and (4) social modeling of pain behavior.

Positive reinforcement of pain behavior refers to the presentation of a stimulus following pain behavior that increases the frequency of the pain behavior in question. A frequently encountered example is pain-contingent attention, which can be especially significant for lonely persons with few meaningful interactions. Medication given p.r.n. for pain and disability payments are other potentially powerful positive reinforcers. Questions about what happens when the patient complains of pain are critical to assessment of this factor.

The avoidance or removal of an aversive stimulus also can increase pain behavior. An example of how avoidance of an aversive stimulus can increase pain behavior would be an older person who develops pain problems that are reinforced by being removed from a situation in which physical or mental deficits are exposed. In many cases the person may have no awareness of the environmental contingencies in question. To assess whether pain behavior may serve as an escape from an aversive stimulus, the behavioral interview would include questions that assess whether or not the patient enjoys or dislikes any activities performed since the onset of pain.

The lack of adequate "well behavior" in a patient's life can pose serious consequences. People who have very few high-quality enjoyable activities in their lives, or who have difficulty coping with the stresses of everyday life, may collapse into a chronic pain problem if injured. The existence of depression may set the stage for the development of maladaptive learned behaviors. Questions about the patient's degree of enjoyment of activities prior to the onset of pain are most likely to yield information about this factor.

Social modeling can be an important factor in the development of pain behavior. Bandura (1971) has found that watching another individual perform a certain behavior increases the probability that the observer will display that behavior. A thorough history that asks about the patient's family or significant others who may have had pain problems may elicit useful information about this type of influence.

Assessment Issues with Stoic Pain

Stoic pain patients differ from doloric patients in that they typically (1) do not respond to environmental factors with an increase in pain behavior, (2) do not demonstrate an increase in pain behavior with the removal of aversive conditions, (3) receive considerable reinforcement of "well" behavior, and (4) do not show pain behavior affected by previous or present social modeling factors. Correlation of activity data with hourly pain level data may be especially useful in assessing stoic patients. A stoic pain condition is suggested by periods of sustained activity without appropriate rest periods, followed by significant increases in subjective pain level coupled with a compensatory decrease in activity level.

Assessment Issues with Assimilated Pain

The assimilated patient manages activity levels and the use of mild analgesics effectively and does not demonstrate learned maladaptive behavioral patterns. These patients usually are seen for clinical conditions other than pain by the primary health-care provider and they may mention pain as a tangential problem. Evidence from a thorough history is likely to show that the patient had good premorbid coping skills and a productive and functional life.

Self-Report Inventories

Minnesota Multiphasic Personality Inventory (MMPI)

The MMPI is used more frequently than any other standardized psychological test in assessing chronic pain patients. It contains ten clinical scales and three validity scales and requires that a patient answer 400 true/false questions. The clinical scales measure the degree to which a person's response pattern differs from the response pattern of the psychiatric patients on whom the test was standardized. The clinical scales of the MMPI are numbered and named as follows: (1) hypochondriasis, (2) depression, (3) hysteria, (4) psychopathic deviance, (5) masculinity–femininity, (6) paranoia, (7) psychasthenia, (8) schizophrenia, (9) hypomania, and (10) social introversion. The three validity scales are listed as scales L, F, and K. They help to indicate whether a person tries to present with fewer or more problems than may be true.

Fordyce (1976) suggests that an effective way to utilize the MMPI when assessing chronic pain patients is to consider patterns of responses as indicating high-frequency or low-frequency behaviors. The utility of this approach is that it seeks to identify maladaptive behavioral patterns, and not less helpful global personality descriptions such as hypochondriasis or hysteria. The essential questions that Fordyce asks from the MMPI are as follows:

1. How ready is a person to signal pain? A high score on scale 1 indicates that the patient probably emits many pain statements.
2. How much does pain behavior cost the person? Elevations on the F scale and scale 2 suggest that the pain has a high emotional cost for the patient or that pain is occurring in someone already having significant emotional distress.
3. Are there other problems for which pain behavior may yield reinforcing time out? Indications of high anxiety (elevations on F, 2, and 7) or of depression (elevations on F and 2 with low scores on 9) suggest long-standing emotional or interpersonal problems.
4. How probable are addiction or habituation to medications? A configuration of scale 1 elevated and higher than scale 2, which is higher than scale 3, suggests that addiction or habituation may be a problem; elevation on scale 4 further supports this hypothesis.
5. How likely is a patient to be responsive to attention or rest? High responsivity is indicated by elevated scores on scales 3, 4, and 9, or low scale 10.
6. How likely are increases in activity to be reinforcing? This assessment is directed toward the patient's energy level, restlessness, and general activity level. The likelihood of a high reinforcement value for activities is suggested by high scales 4 and 9, or high K with high scales 2 and 7.

Using the MMPI to predict response to treatment has not yielded definitive results (McCreary et al. 1979). This lack of consistency in assessment underlines the necessity for using more than just an MMPI for prediction.

Nevertheless, the MMPI is a useful tool that can generate hypotheses that then can be tested against data from other pain assessment procedures. Some of the hypotheses that are suggested by it can be rather subtle and not immediately obtained from other sources.

One of the main criticisms of the MMPI is that it was developed for a psychiatric population and not for a medical population. Recent authors have sought to remedy this shortcoming by developing paper-and-pencil tests specifically for pain patients.

McGill Pain Questionnaire

The McGill Pain Questionnaire (Melzack, 1975) was developed to assess chronic pain patients and consists of three classes of words that patients use to describe the subjective qualities of their pain experience (Fig. 9-1). The descriptive words relate to either sensory, affective, or evaluative aspects of the pain experience. One advantage of the McGill questionnaire is that it provides quantifiable data on pain intensity that can be used for research purposes. It also provides a fairly specific understanding of the subjective quality of the patient's pain. Information from the sensory class of words can be used to double-check other subjective estimates of pain, such as the rating obtained from a visual analog scale. One of

PAIN QUESTIONNAIRE

Some of the words below describe your *present* pain. Circle *ONLY* those words that best describe it. Leave out any category that is not suitable. Use only a single word in each appropriate category — the one that applies best.

1
Flickering
Quivering
Pulsing
Throbbing
Beating
Pounding

2
Jumping
Flashing
Shooting

3
Pricking
Boring
Drilling
Stabbing
Lancinating

4
Sharp
Cutting
Lacerating

5
Pinching
Pressing
Gnawing
Cramping
Crushing

6
Tugging
Pulling
Wrenching

7
Hot
Burning
Scalding
Searing

8
Tingling
Itchy
Smarting
Stinging

9
Dull
Sore
Hurting
Aching
Heavy

10
Tender
Taut
Rasping
Splitting

11
Tiring
Exhausting

12
Sickening
Suffocating

13
Fearful
Frightful
Terrifying

14
Punishing
Gruelling
Cruel
Vicious
Killing

15
Wretched
Blinding

16
Annoying
Troublesome
Miserable
Intense
Unbearable

17
Spreading
Radiating
Penetrating
Piercing

18
Tight
Numb
Drawing
Squeezing
Tearing

19
Cool
Cold
Freezing

20
Nagging
Nauseating
Agonizing
Dreadful
Torturing

FIG. 9-1. McGill pain questionnaire

the major difficulties with the McGill is that some of the words that are used in the instrument are not readily understood by many pain patients.

Millon Behavioral Health Inventory (MBHI).

The MBHI is a recently developed self-report inventory that contains 150 true/false questions (Millon et al., 1979). It was designed to provide information about a wide range of measures important in assessment and decision making in a variety of medical settings. The first section contains scales that assess major personality styles important in determining responses in medical situations. A second section assesses attitudes about health and different sources and levels of psychosocial stresses. A third set of scales assesses whether or not a patient's response to the illness has been substantially complicated by psychological, social, or environmental factors. The fourth and final section contains prognostic indices that seek to predict patient response to treatment for several medical conditions, including chronic pain. Because the instrument was developed on a medical population rather than a psychiatric population, it may have greater clinical utility than the MMPI, but additional research must be performed in order to document its effectiveness with pain patients.

Patient Pain Drawings

Pain drawings are another form of paper-and-pencil self-report that have been useful in assessment. The patient is asked to indicate on a silhouette drawing the location and quality of the pain. The drawing can be viewed as a sample of pain behavior; those patients who indicate extensive pain involvement over multiple locations and utilize multiple adjectives to describe their pain are those who tend to have the most maladaptive learned behavioral patterns and are most likely to have doloric pain. By using these drawings, Mooney and colleagues (1976) found that they were able to pick with 75 percent accuracy those patients whose eventual work-up indicated a significant emotional involvement in their pain problem. The interpretation of pain drawings, however, is essentially subjective and therefore may have significant limitations.

Activity Diary

An activity diary is a self-report of the person's daily activities. A commonly used type of activity diary asks the patient to record on an hourly basis how much time is spent reclining, sitting, or standing/walking (Fig. 9-2). If the patient shows more than 80 hours per week in the latter two categories combined, but still indicates difficulty in managing pain, then a stoic pain condition may be present. A doloric patient would be expected to be reinforced by rest, and therefore would be likely to have less than 80 hours per week of uptime.

Visual Analog Scales

Visual analog scales are designed to measure the subjective intensity of pain. The scale is a straight line, the ends of which are defined as the extreme limits of the patient's pain experience (Fig. 9-3). The instrument is useful in that, like the McGill, it quantifies the pain experience and thus can be used for research

ACTIVITY DIARY

Day of Week: ______________________ **Date:** ______________________

	SITTING		WALKING/STANDING		RECLINING	
	Major Activity	Time	Major Activity	Time	Major Activity	Time
Midnight 12-1						
1-2						
2-3						
3-4						
4-5						
5-6 A.M.						
6-7						
7-8						
8-9						
9-10						
10-11						
11-12						
12-1 Noon						
1-2						
2-3						
3-4						
4-5						
5-6 P.M.						
6-7						
7-8						
8-9						
9-10						
10-11						
11-12						
TOTAL						

FIG. 9-2. Activity Diary

purposes. The effectiveness of treatment with a particular patient can be assessed by repeated administrations of the form as treatment progresses. Information from hourly pain recordings can be compared with information from an activity diary and medication records. This comparison may yield relationships between activity levels or medication usage and pain levels.

PAIN INTENSITY RATING

Name: ____________________ **Date Form Filled Out:** __________

At any given point in time, we would like for you to think of your pain intensity as falling somewhere *between* having no pain (0%, lowest point) up to having pain "as bad as it could be" (100%, highest point).

Please estimate your *average* pain intensity over the last week by making a vertical (up and down) mark I somewhere along the line below. This will give us an estimate of your *general* pain intensity.

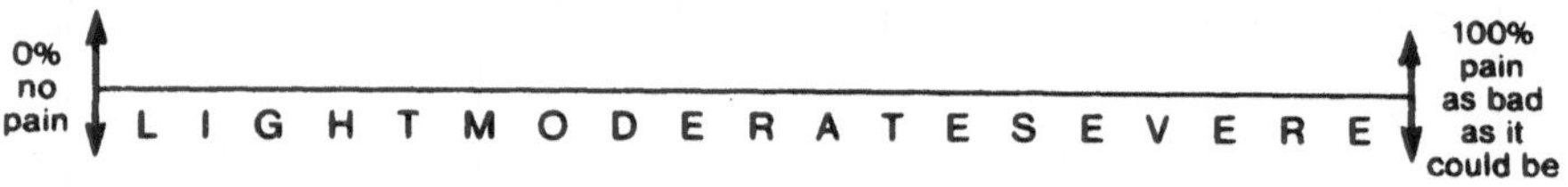

FIG. 9-3. Visual analog scale

Two problems that beset any paper-and-pencil psychological test, regardless of the quality of its construction, are that the information obtained may reflect patients' judgment of how they should respond, and that what they believe to be true about themselves may be different from their actual behavior. Thus, self-report inventories should not be used as the sole source of psychological information.

Submaximum Effort Tourniquet Technique

The submaximum effort tourniquet technique (SETT) is a psychophysiological procedure that assesses the reaction of a patient to an experimentally induced pain state (Smith et al., 1966). The typical procedure is to restrict blood flow in a patient's nondominant arm via a tourniquet until a state of tolerance is reached. Sternbach et al. (1974) extended the use of the procedure to chronic pain patients by asking them to indicate when the ischemic pain was equivalent to their clinical pain and also when they had reached tolerance. Sternbach and his associates suggested that the ratio of the clinical equivalent time divided by time to tolerance (the tourniquet ratio) may be useful in determining subjective pain intensity. Comparison of this ratio with the patient's rating of subjective pain intensity on a visual analog scale may indicate whether the patient tends to exaggerate or inhibit pain expressions.

The SETT, however, has not been as robust a clinical tool as had been hoped. One of the primary difficulties has been that the tourniquet ratio assumes a linear relationship between elapsed time in the ischemic condition and increases in pain. Fox and colleagues (1979) found that only three of 27 subjects (11 percent) demonstrated a linear relationship between pain estimate and elapsed time. This assessment tool, however, does merit continued evaluation in that it is an actual assessment of the behavior in question, that is, a patient's behavioral response to pain.

INTEGRATION OF INFORMATION

A solid understanding of the theoretical framework from which these assessment procedures have been developed is necessary in order to utilize effectively the assessment tools discussed in this chapter. The interested reader is referred to the cited references for additional background information. Additionally, specific training in a pain management clinic with a colleague who specializes in behavioral assessment methods may be highly useful to the practitioner without formal training in this area.

Treatment modalities must be carefully chosen on the basis of assessment results. Some chronic pain treatment programs utilize almost any and all treatment procedures that hold promise of working without accurately assessing the unique facets of each patient's problem. The use of a "shotgun" approach such as this offers little possibility for advancing the state of knowledge in pain treatment because, without accurate assessment, it is impossible to determine which aspects of a program are especially useful for certain types of patients.

The primary task of the diagnostician is, of course, to integrate the collected data into a consistent understanding of the patient. A sound assessment is probable if information from a patient's history, medical evaluation, and psychological evaluation suggest the same conclusion. Conversely, if conclusions that have been developed based on historical information or medical evaluation are not supported by psychological data, then it is incumbent upon the investigator to sort through the available data and discover the reason for the discrepancy.

FUTURE DIRECTIONS

Recent research in psychology has considered the role that cognitions play in the pain experience. Meichenbaum (1977) has suggested that assessment procedures profitably would include a "cognitive-functional" analysis. Such an analysis considers overt influences (environmental factors) and the influence of covert factors (a person's cognitions) on the experience of pain. The observation that a person's thoughts can have a profound affect on a subjective experience such as pain is not new, but little research exists in the area. Bookwalter et al. (1978) describe a conceptual grid that analyzes the pain experience in terms of communication to one's self and others (Fig. 9-4). A patient is asked to complete a self-report checklist with 20 items in each of the four categories listed on Figure 9-4. The relative frequency of responses in each of the four areas allows the diagnostician to determine if the patient acknowledges high levels of pain-related communication to self (thoughts) or others, and if nonverbal communication may be a significant factor in the patient's pain experience. Research with this and other instruments that consider the role of cognitive factors in pain assessment is still in the preliminary stage, but may add one more piece to our understanding of the complex puzzle of pain.

Assessment protocols that predict whether a patient with acute pain is at a high risk to develop a chronic pain problem are needed. Epidemiological research could have profound effects on health care delivery for pain patients. Many patients who are seen in a chronic pain center would not need "comprehensive pain management" if accurately assessed and treated soon after the onset of a pain problem.

Because few centers for chronic pain management utilize the same assessment protocols, communication between centers and treatment outcome comparisons are difficult. The development of more standardized and objective psychological procedures may help to alleviate this problem.

Pain Behavior is Whatever I Think, Say, or Do That Communicates to Myself or Others That I am Experiencing Pain.

		COMMUNICATION	
		With Others	With Myself
BEHAVIOR	Non-Verbal Behavior (what I do)	(1) Those things I do (i.e., my behaviors or actions) that communicate to other people that I am experiencing pain.	(2) Those things I do (i.e., my behaviors or actions) that by my doing them I communicate to myself that I am experiencing pain
	Verbal Behavior (what I think or say)	(3) Those things that I say that communicate to other people that I am experiencing pain	(4) Those thoughts or things I say to myself that communicate to myself that I am experiencing pain

FIG. 9-4. Conceptual grid for assessment of chronic pain behavior

REFERENCES

Bandura, A. 1971. Analysis of modeling processes. In *Psychological Modeling: Conflicting Theories,* A. Bandura (Ed.). Chicago: Aldine/Atherton, pp. 6–62.

Bookwalter, S.T., Johnson, S.J., and Volkerts, P. 1978. A conceptual grid for the assessment of chronic pain behavior. *Arch. Phys. Med. Rehab.* 59:327.

Fordyce, W. 1976. *Behavioral Methods for Chronic Pain and Illness.* St. Louis: C.V. Mosby.

Fordyce, W.E., Brana, S.F., Holcomb, R.J., et al. 1978. Relationship of patient sematic pain descriptions to physician diagnostic judgments, activity level measures, and MMPI. *Pain* 5:293–303.

Fox, C.D., Steger, H.G., and Jennison, J.H. 1979. Ratio scaling of pain perception with the submaximum effort tourniquet technique. *Pain* 7:21–29.

McCreary, C., Turner, J., and Dawson, E. 1979. The MMPI as a predictor of response to conservative treatment for low back pain. *J. Clin. Psychol.* 35:278–284.

Meichenbaum, D. 1977. *Cognitive-Behavior Modification.* New York: Plenum Press.

Melzack, R. 1973. *The Puzzle of Pain.* Harmondsworth, England: Penguin Books.

Melzack, R. 1975. The McGill pain questionnaire: Major properties and scoring methods. *Pain* 1:277–299.

Millon, T., Green, C.J., and Meagher, R.D. 1979. The MBHI: A new inventory for the psychodiagnostician in medical settings. *Prof. Psychol.* 10:529–539.

Mooney, V., Cairns, D., and Robertson, J. 1976. A system for evaluating and treating chronic back disability. *West. J. Med.* 124:370–376.

Smith, G.M., Egbert, L.D., Markowitz, R.A., et al. 1966. An experimental pain method sensitive to morphine in man: The submaximum effort tourniquet technique. *J. Pharmacol. Therap.* 154:324–332.

Steger, H.G., Fox, C.D., and Feinberg, S.D. 1980. Behavioral evaluation and management of chronic pain. In *Behavior and the Disabled: Assessment and Management,* D.S. Bishop (Ed.). Baltimore: Williams & Wilkins.

Sternbach, R.A., Murphy, R.W., Timmermans, G., et al. 1974. Measuring the severity of clinical pain. In *Advances in Neurology,* J.J. Bonica, (Ed.). New York: Raven Press, pp. 281–288.

Wolff, B.B. 1978. Behavioral measurement of human pain. In *The Psychology of Pain,* R. Sternbach, (Ed.). New York: Raven Press, pp. 129–168.

The author appreciates the review of this chapter by Drs. Herbert Steger and Corey Fox.

10

The Medical Diagnostic Process

STEVEN F. BRENA

Changes of biomedical functions are not by themselves reliable indicators in the diagnosis of chronic pain states. Diagnostic assessment of chronic pain is a multidimensional measurement task. Various techniques of assessment are briefly discussed. The Emory Pain Estimate Model for pain quantification and classification is described and supportive data are presented. Techniques for vocational and disability evaluation for pain-disabled patients and data concerning the relationship of chronic pain states to impairment and disability are presented.

Changes of biomedical functions often are viewed as good diagnostic indicators of a systemic disease process; for instance, blood levels of oxygen, carbon dioxide, and lactates are abnormal when the respiratory system is impaired. A satisfactory biological indicator for pain would be a measurable body function that is consistently present or increased when pain is perceived and absent or decreased when pain is not perceived.

No reliable biological pain indicator is presently available. Current research efforts are focusing on peptide levels in the spinal fluid and in the blood as possible physiological monitors of an acute painful perception. However, research findings in the field of nociceptive physiology are puzzling and seem to raise questions more than to provide answers; the application of such research in clinical practice is still merely a hope for the future. Moreover, chronicity always fosters the onset of multiple accidental factors that may affect the painful experience with little cause-and-effect relationship to biomedical findings. Thus chronic pain cannot be diagnosed adequately solely within the framework of the biomedical model. To assume that a painful state of long duration can be "cured" by the removal of any pathological abnormality is an oversimplification that may lead to random rather than to scientifically predictable results.

THE MEASUREMENT OF PAIN

Every diagnostic process is a form of measurement and must be based on measurement techniques. The diagnostic process in chronic pain involves a formidable multidimensional measurement task. Though the quantification of clinical pain traditionally has rested on the postulate that the patient's verbal report is a reliable index, several studies have shown that pain complaints may be "learned language" dependent on variables other than nociceptive perceptions (Agnew & Mersky, 1976; Bailey & Davidson, 1976; Melzack & Torgerson, 1971). This complexity is underscored by the findings of Fordyce et al. (1978), who demonstrated that even when using the same set of data, physicians' judgments as to organic versus nonorganic pain show only moderate levels of reliability.

Early work done on the measurement of pain focused mainly on measurable pain thresholds in response to quantified electrical, thermal, or mechanical stimuli. Historically the best known of such methods is the dolorimeter designed by Hardy et al. (1940). More recently Sternbach et al. (1974) have designed the tourniquet test, which is a newer technique for measuring the severity of clinical pain, based partially on the threshold model. This test is described in Chapter 9 of this book.

Winnie et al. (1974) have presented a method of pain classification that includes the use of differential neural blocking. Following lumbar puncture, normal saline, 0.25 percent procaine, 0.5 percent procaine, and 1 percent procaine are injected at ten-minute intervals. Relief following saline injection is interpreted as placebo response or as an indication of "psychogenic mechanisms"; relief after 0.25 percent procaine with no sensory loss is labeled "sympathetic pain"; relief after 0.5 percent or 0.1 percent procaine is interpreted as "somatic pain"; no relief of pain despite anesthesia and motor blockade is indication of "central pain" or malingering. The reliability and the validity of the Winne method are highly questionable, because the technique is based on patients' verbal responses and physicians' interpretation of those responses.

On none of the above studies has there been a systematic attempt to obtain a quantified assessment of stimulus intensity (in terms of pathological findings) of pain responses, and of correlates between these two sets of data. Few attempts have been made to construct reliable methods of quantification and classification of chronic pain states based on measurable data different from the patient's verbal reports alone.

Black and Chapman (1976) did provide a quantified assessment of pain by devising a three-factor index using estimates of patients' somatic input, anxiety, and depression (SAD). The patient's total suffering is represented by the vector sum of these three factors. The authors themselves recognized the limitation of the SAD index, which fails to incorporate relevant ecological factors.

Duncan et al. (1978) have designed a computer-based pain profile for classification of each patient, which is based on a mathematical comparison of three indices representing various pain dimensions. The organic index represents the summation of objective evidence of organic pathologic problems. Measured by the clinician on a 0–1.00 severity scale using routine diagnostic methods, it includes three compartments of morbidity: (1) systemic disorders, (2) neurologic disorders, and (3) nonneurologic disorders within the painful region. The psychosocial index considers several different factors, including (1) life stresses and (2) degrees of *formal* psychopathology. Measurement of these factors is achieved through several paper-and-pencil questionnaires. The pain behavior index considers the perceptual-discriminative and affective-motivational aspects of chronic pain. Measurements are obtained via the McGill Pain Questionnaire, global pain estimates of percent pain severity, the Sternbach tourniquet pain-matching test, and assessments of drug abuse, abuse of pain therapy, and the degree of functional impairment.

The pain profile described by Duncan et al. is accurate and comprehensive, but time consuming for both the patient and the practicing physician. The authors themselves recognize that their pain profile is mostly a research tool and a teaching model, but express hope that it eventually may direct primary care clinicians toward a more thorough appreciation of chronic pain patients.

THE EMORY PAIN ESTIMATE MODEL

Brena and Koch (1975) at Emory University have designed a pain estimate model (Fig. 10-1), for classification and quantification of chronic pain states, which is based on the analysis of three quantifiable sets of data: (1) measures of organic pathology, (2) measures of illness behavior, and (3) the relationship between pathology–behavior correlates, expressed in four different classes of chronic pain states. The following assessments are made.

Physician-Based Pathology Assessment

On the basis of all available medical data, the observed pathology is rated on a horizontal, continuous severity scale from 0 to 10. Up to 2.5 points are assigned on this scale for evidence of pathology on each of the followng sets of data: (1) physical examination, (2) neurological testing, (3) radiological studies, and (4) laboratory tests.

Patient-Based Pain Assessment

Each patient routinely is given a paper-and-pencil testing packet, which includes (1) measures of subjective pain intensity, including a visual-analog 0–100 scale on which the patient rates pain intensity, and the McGill Questionnaire, on which the patient selects words representing different levels of pain intensity; (2) an activity record on which the patient records daily the amount of time spent

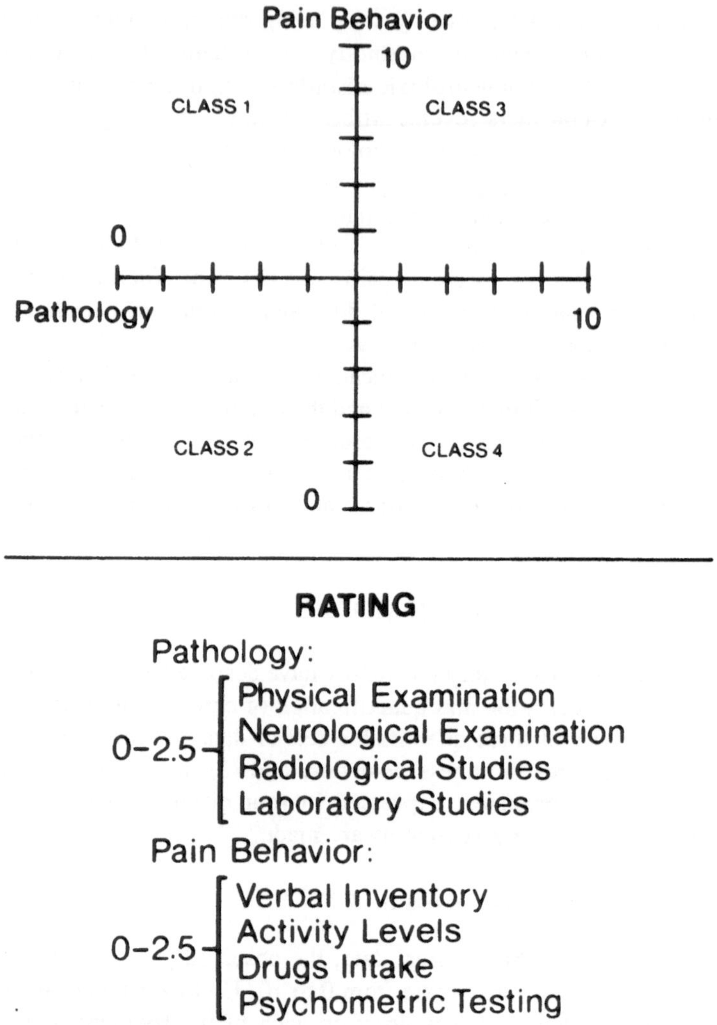

FIG. 10-1. The Emory Pain Estimate Model

participating in activities of daily living (ADL); (3) a medication record; and (4) the Minnesota Multiphasic Personality Inventory (MMPI). In each of these four types of measures, up to 2.5 points are assigned, depending upon the degree of pain verbalization, activity, drug misuse, and personality maladjustment. This assessment yields a measure of pain behavior ranging from 0 to 10 on a vertical scale.

Classes of Pain

From the assessment of pathology and pain behavior, patients are divided into four classes of chronic pain states. In Class I, pain behavior scores are high (5 or above) and pathology scores are low (below 5). In Class II the patients score low on both sets of variables. In Class III pathology and behavior scores are both high. In Class IV pathology scores are high and behavior scores are low. Assignment of 15 case histories to classes by five independent physicians yielded a Pearson product–moment correlation of 0.85, indicating a high reliability for the model (Brena et al., 1976). This high agreement is possible because the model provides an easy method to weigh the physical data that the physician habitually employs in his/her daily practice against the behavioral data that can be obtained through the use of a few simple questionnaires. The result is an operational definition of a pain patient, which any physician can clearly understand and communicate.

The diagnostic value of the Emory Pain Estimate Model for practical purposes is obvious. Class I patients are "pain amplifiers"; despite low pathology ratings, they are pain-disabled with low activity levels, prominent ecological stressors, and misuse of several drugs, including central analgesics and sedatives on a p.r.n. schedule. These conditioned illness behaviors often are strengthened by various socioeconomic rewards. A commonly encountered example of a Class I pain patient would be the pain-disabled injured worker, with chronic low back pain and low pathology. Class I pain patients are not likely to improve following traditional biomedical management, which may actually reinforce their sick roles. On the contrary they are good candidates for pain control and rehabilitation programs for drug detoxification and physical and emotional readjustment.

Class II patients are "pain verbalizers" characterized by highly dramatized pain complaints with ill-defined anatomical patterns. Despite their complaints such patients are still functional with close to normal ADL, no misuse of depressant medications, and various states of neuroticism on MMPI scales. A good example of a Class II pain patient would be a middle-aged, normally functioning housewife with chronic pelvic pain and low pathology, gulping down several Tylenol and vitamin pills and showing a "conversion V" profile on the MMPI. Proper management of Class II pain patients must be designed to keep them functional despite continuous complaining, through directive counseling and placebo medication. Unwise use of central analgesics, sedatives, and antianxiety agents; unnecessary hospitalization; and poorly documented exploratory surgery are likely to transfer Class II patients into Class I with no other result than to increase the cost of their medical care and produce the need for disability benefits.

Class III pain patients are "chronic sufferers" with clear evidence of biomedical findings on standard medical investigations and high-intensity illness behavior. However, these two variables are independent so that the resolution of pathological problems is not necessarily followed by an extinction of illness behavior. An example of a Class III patient would be a cancer patient whose malignancy has been checked and stabilized but who continues to grow more dysfunctional physically and emotionally. Class III patients often need traditional medical treatment for their pathological problem matched with pain control and rehabilitation management.

Class IV pain patients are "pain reducers." They are able to contain their illness behavior despite the presence of well-documented organic disease.

The high percentage of patients assigned to Class I (pain-disabled) and Class II (high pain verbalizers) with minimal evidence of pathology clearly indicates the importance of learning factors in chronic pain (see Table 10-1).

DISABILITY EVALUATION

At present, health and legal professionals, insurance companies, industry, government, and the patients themselves are faced with a system of disability evaluation that is chaotic at best. The patient may find differences from physician to physician, state to state, and agency to agency. All parties involved are currently forced to make judgments on an inadequate information base and the outcome often depends upon who has chosen the best attorney rather than who has the most substantial claim. Disability awards often are granted to those who have learned to play the best "pain game" rather than those who have objective data.

No system of evaluation will avoid controversy, but the better the information upon which decisions are made, the fairer the decisions will be. A comprehensive evaluation of a physically impaired patient must (1) review the medical status, (2) assess the illness behavior, (3) establish a pain classification,

Table 10-1.
Emory Pain Estimate Model Pain Classification

Class	Workers' Compensation	No Paid Disability
	(N = 74)	(N = 70)
I	72%	40%
II	0%	35%
III	28%	21%
IV	0%	3%

(4) provide an impairment and disability rating, (5) match potential for work to possible vocations, and (6) provide a specific judgment as to the disability for a specific job.

Steps 1, 2, and 3 are part of the diagnostic process involved in the Emory Pain Estimate Model. An impairment rating can be made based on the well-known American Medical Association's (AMA) guidelines. While the AMA guidelines are imperfect and not entirely accurate, they are a widely used standard. The definition of disability involves a multitude of factors, such as motor performance, motivation, discomfort, and fatigue. For example, a left upper extremity amputee may be 100 percent disabled as a violinist, but not disabled as a radio or television announcer. The disability rating therefore requires comprehensive vocational testing. No vocational evaluation system can be expected to assess completely every facet of disability; however, of the many systems that have been developed to evaluate disability, two appear to be emerging as leaders in the field: the Hester System and the Valpar System.

The Hester System is a computerized method of assessing a person's vocational abilities. It consists of 27 factor-pure tests such as manual dexterity, coordination and perception. After testing the raw scores and some additional characteristics about the individual are fed into a computer. The computer analyzes the individual scores to determine how his/her abilities relate to those jobs contained in the *Dictionary of Occupational Titles*. General categories and some specific categories of jobs are listed on the computer printout as being very feasible, feasible, or nonfeasible for the patient. Testing according to the Hester System takes about five hours to complete.

The Valpar System is an individual evaluation process that gathers data on cognitive and psychomotor abilities and on interest and achievement. Testing consists of several work samples from which traits are measured that are universal in nature and are related to a person's success in many occupations. Examples of these samples include Clerical Comprehension and Aptitude, Multilevel Sorting, Simulated Assembly, and Soldering and Inspection (Electronics). An advantage of the Valpar System over the Hester is that it uses a specified individualized evaluation plan for each evaluee, based on an attempt to reproduce actual work situations. It takes about eight hours to complete the testing. The system shows a test–retest reliability coefficient for each of the various component work samples ranging from 0.85 to 0.97.

Example of Comprehensive Disability Evaluation

Patient A.B. is a former mechanic with chronic low back pain of three years' duration, following a back sprain suffered on the job. He has been receiving Workers' Compensation benefits and has been out of work since the injury. The Emory Pain Estimate Model has placed him in Class I with a pathology level of

3.5 and a behavior level of 7.1. Impairment rating of the whole body is assessed as 5 percent. The Hester printout shows various jobs requiring the skills of a mechanic to be "very feasible." The diagnosis is learned illness behavior in excess of biomedical findings. The patient is not a candidate for further disability benefits. He should be directed to return to gainful employment promptly, possibly through a brief period of vocational training to ease him back into the labor force after three years of inactivity.

Brena et al. (1979) have studied relationships of chronic pain states to impairment and disability. Out of 101 patients sampled, 60 were assigned to Class I, 16 to Class II, 25 to Class III, and none to Class IV. Consistent with the predictions, higher levels of both physical pathology and pain behavior were significantly related to higher levels of both impairment and disability. Class I patients showed a higher impairment and disability rating than Class II patients, whereas Class III patients showed the highest impairment and disability scores. The finding that 59 percent of these patients showed higher disability than impairment ratings relates partially to the different definitions of impairment and disability; many of these patients were blue collar workers whose jobs involved heavy manual labor. However, a disability rating significantly higher than the impairment rating clearly implies the possibility of gainful employment in other jobs that are less demanding. To grant blanket disability to Class I pain patients with low impairment is socially irresponsible and medically wrong, because it condemns these individuals to a life-style of learned illness and hopelessness. The findings of this study further support the extreme need of careful evaluation of pain states, impairment, and disability in cases where litigation is pending.

APPENDIX

At the 1980 meeting of the American Pain Society (New York, September 5–7) several reports indicated that infrared thermography may be of value in the diagnosis of chronic pain states mostly to differentiate psychogenic (learned) and organic (pathogenic) pain. According to these studies (Liao; Uematsu & Long; Goodley) the anatomical area of pain location shows a lower level of infrared radiation than the unaffected contralateral side. In one study (Liao), an increase in infrared radiation was demonstrated in the painful region following acupuncture treatment.

The infrared radiation displayed by thermography is primarily a function of vascular flow. If this technique is proved to be reliable and valid, it may offer an excellent qualitative method for assessment of nociceptive abnormality. Of course, the technique will give no informaton about the other dimensions of chronic pain. Moreover, because thermograms are a function of blood flow, the question about whether these blood flow changes may represent organic vascular changes or emotional arousal expressed through vasomotor disturbances will remain unanswered.

REFERENCES

Agnew, D.C., and Merskey, H. 1976. Words of chronic pain. *Pain* 2:73–82.

Bailey, C. and Davidson, P. 1976. The language of pain intensity. *Pain* 2:319–324.

Black, R.G., and Chapman, C.R. 1976. The S.A.D. index for clinical assessment of pain. In *Advances in Pain Research and Therapy*, J.J. Bonica and D. Albe-Fessard. (Eds.) New York: Raven Press, pp. 301–305.

Brena, S.F., Chapman, S.L., Stegall, P.G., and Chyatte, S.B. 1979. Chronic pain states: Their relationship to impairment and disability. *Arch. Phys. Med. Rehab.* 60:387–389.

Brena, S.F., and Koch, D.L. 1975. The "Pain Estimate" for quantification and classification of chronic pain states. *Anesthesiol. Rev.* 2:8–13.

Brena, S.F., Koch, D.L., and Moss, R.M. 1976. Reliability of the pain estimate model. *Anesthesiol. Rev.* 3:28–29.

Duncan, G.H., Gregg, J.M., and Ghia, J.N. 1978. The pain profile: A computerized system for assessment of chronic pain. *Pain* 5:275–284.

Fordyce, W.E., Brena, S.F., Holcomb, R., et al. 1978. Relationship of semantic pain descriptions to physician diagnostic judgments, activity level measures, and MMPI. *Pain* 5:293–303.

Goodley, P.H. 1980. Musculoskeletal pain and thermography. Presentation at the Second Meeting of the American Pain Society, New York, Sept. 5.

Hardy, J.D., Wolff, H.G., Goodell, H. 1940. Studies on pain: A new method for measuring pain threshold. *J. Clin. Invest.* 19:649–662.

Liao, S.J. 1980. Thermography for chronic pain and acupuncture. Presentation at the Second Meeting of the American Pain Society, New York, Sept. 5.

Melzack, R., and Torgerson, W.S. 1971. On the language of pain. *Anesthesiology* 34:50–59.

Sternbach, R.A., Murphy, R.W., Timmermans, G., and Greenhoot, J.H. 1974. Measuring the severity of clinical pain. In *Advances in Neurology*, J.J. Bonica (Ed.) New York: Raven Press, pp. 281–288.

Uematsu, S. and Long, D. 1980. Thermography in the differential diagnosis of reflex sympathetic dystrophy and "psychogenic pain." Presentation at the Second Meeting of the American Pain Society, New York, Sept. 5.

Winnie, A.P., Ramamurthy, S., and Durrani, Z. 1974. Diagnostic and therapeutic nerve blocks: Recent advances and techniques. In *Advances in Neurology*, J.J. Bonica. (Ed.) New York: Raven Press, pp. 455–460.

11

An Algorithm for Decision-Making in Patients with Pain

STEVEN F. BRENA and STANLEY L. CHAPMAN

Wisdom and sound judgment are required in the diagnostic and therapeutic approach to patients with pain, so as to avoid needless medical interventions for diagnosis and therapy. An algorithm for graded decision making in patients with pain is presented. Two levels of practice are considered, each one consisting of several steps, directed toward the goal of returning the patient to a state of health. A "salvage protocol" for patients who fail with treatment is proposed.

The goal of every health professional, as he/she approaches the patient with pain, is to return that patient to a state of health, as defined by the World Health Organization (Chapter 2), and not merely to correct and remove any identifiable disease process. In the pursuit of this goal, the practitioner is bound by a code of ethics expressed as the rule *Primum Non Nocere*, which warns that his/her first duty is to avoid harm to the patient physically, emotionally, or economically.

Because of its complexity, the diagnosis of pain problems heavily taxes the clinical acumen of every practitioner, often driving him/her into recommending sophisticated, expensive tests and possibly overabundant hospitalizations for diagnostic procedures. Modern technology has allowed such extensive biological investigation that it is likely that physiological abnormality could be found in almost every healthy individual. The question no longer is what to do in order to reach a correct diagnosis, but how much should be done to achieve the goal at reasonable cost and with minimal risk of harming the patient. In the face of all of this medical technology, sound clinical judgments thus are needed badly. Diagnostic procedures should be used to answer specific questions in a step-by-step ordered sequence. An algorithm for decision making in patients with pain drawn from eight years' experience is thus proposed as a way to organize thought processes about the management of the patient with pain (Fig. 11-1).

The *Encyclopedia Brittanica* defines an algorithm as "a set of steps designed to achieve a complex *mathematical* operation, each step carrying the

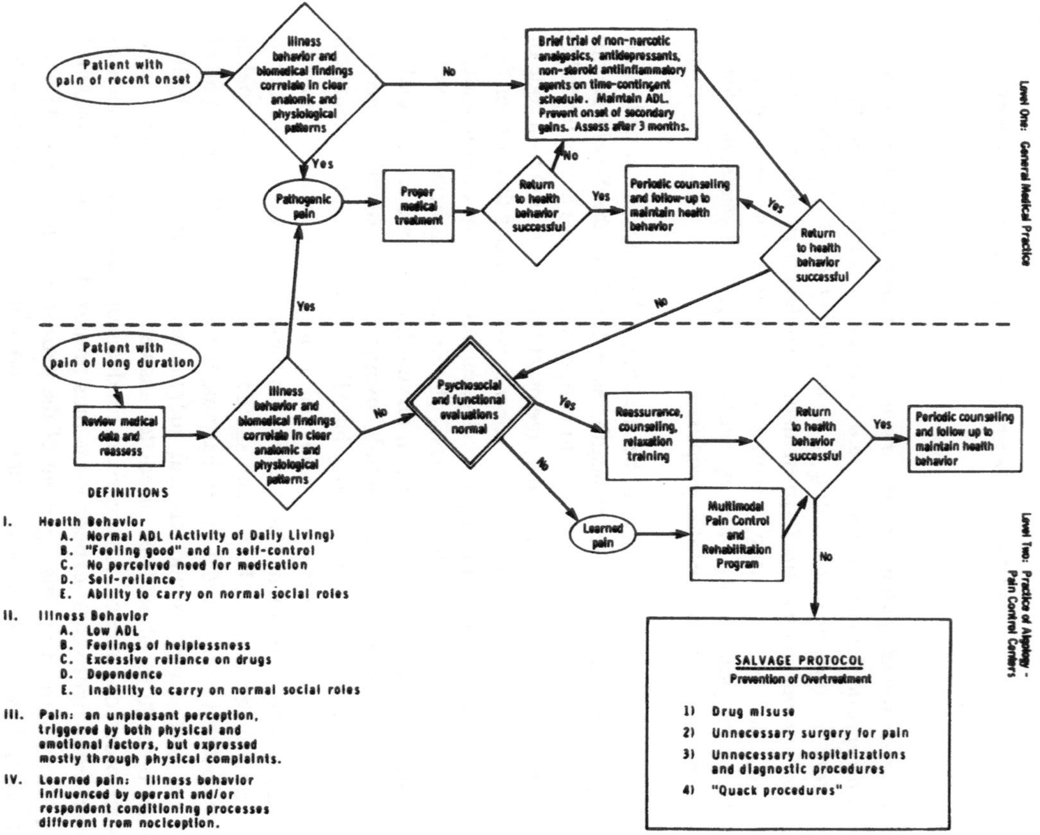

FIG. 11-1. Emory algorithm for decision making in patients with pain from: Brena, S.F., and Chapman, S.L. 1982. "Chronic pain: An algorithm for management." Post. Grad. Med. 72; 111:117

operation forward by one small increment and perhaps with a built-in repetition of a step . . . until certain conditions are reached''.

For the purpose of the Emory Pain Algorithm, the following symbols have been chosen: diamond-shaped signs = decision points; oval-shaped signs = diagnoses; rectangular signs = treatment strategies.

Pathogenic Pain Versus Learned Pain

The first crucial step in the algorithm is to identify the nature of the pain problem. Is it a primary biological symptom or a set of conditioned behaviors? The time factor alone is not of great value. Pain complaints from a recent injury or disease may be learned responses based on previous similar experiences and painful perceptions from a chronic disease may still be symptoms of primary biological significance. A likely example of the first case would be a worker with high-intensity complaints of low back pain from a recent on-the-job lumbar sprain, who has returned to work following a period of paid disability from a previous work-related accident. A good example of the second case would be a fully functional osteoarthritic patient with pathogenic pain from degenerative joint disease. The algorithm recognizes two levels of practice in the management of pain problems: (1) pathogenic pain is the field of traditional medical practice, where the detection and correction of pertinent pathological factors should lead toward returns to states of health; (2) learned pain is the field of algology, where diagnostic teamwork and multimodal rehabilitation programs should provide similar results.

Independent analysis of biomedical findings and illness behaviors is of key diagnostic value. In everyday office practice, a ''subjective pain profile'' can be obtained easily from the patient's pain description, and from the observation of the patient's gait, posture, facial expression, attitude, and affect. An ''objective pain profile'' also can be obtained by mapping possible nociceptive factors from a conventional medical examination. Finally, a ''social pain profile'' can be constructed through simple questions about the social milieu of the patients and its perceived impact upon the painful experience. In most cases the entire office investigation should not take longer than 30 minutes if well organized in a routine procedure with the use of data-base sheets (see the appendix).

Level 1

If the subjective and objective pain profiles match significantly in clear anatomical and physiological terms, a diagnosis of pathogenic pain is likely. Class IV patients of the Emory Pain Estimate Model belong to this group. In cases of frank pathogenic pain, further in-depth diagnostic investigation is well justified to identify correctly the biological disorder and eventually to correct it.

From this step on, a variety of algorithms could be constructed to guide the clinician in decision making for every known disease entity.

On the other hand, if subjective and objective profiles do not correlate well and/or the social profile shows suspicious evidence of socioeconomic factors on which illness behavior may be contingent, a more conservative approach should be followed. Hospitalization and conventional diagnostic tests should be limited to a minimum, mostly to rule out potentially lethal pathology. For instance, a patient in this group with primary back pain of very recent onset may be given a technetium bone scan to rule out a tumor and/or inflammatory disease of the spine, but should be spared myelograms and other neurological tests for disc disease.

At Level 1 of pain management, a main concern is prevention of learned illness behaviors. This task may be accomplished through various steps: avoid medication "p.r.n. for pain" and the prescription of opiates, central analgesics, sedatives, and antianxiety agents in the functional, ambulatory patient (see Chapter 12); restore activity as soon as possible after the resolution of the acute disease process or surgery; explain the role of normal activities of daily living in preserving a physiological and emotional state of well being; discourage sick roles and emphasize the rewards of health behavior. Relatives may be educated to cooperate in this task. Such simple guidelines are not time consuming and are well within the feasibility of an average office practice.

In tracing the history of many unjustified disability cases, where disability compensation was granted to patients with little evidence of actual pathological findings, it has been found that quite often the first step in the direction of the disability claim was an open-ended disability statement by a clinician who unknowingly rubber-stamped the patient's own desire to avoid work through high-intensity pain complaints (Florence, 1979). Any statement of disability should be well documented and time limited. To emphasize this crucial point, it is useful to repeat that an unjustified disability involves an average waste in excess of $20,000 per year to the taxpayer.

Level 2

At this level pain management is concerned with the classification and the rehabilitation of patients with learned pain, who show one or more of the "five D's," those groups of symptoms discussed in Chapter 1 and summarized here:

1. Dramatization in describing the painful experience—vague, diffuse, inconsistent complaints with no known anatomical and physiological patterns
2. Drug misuse
3. Dysfunction—various bodily impairments from physical and emotional factors

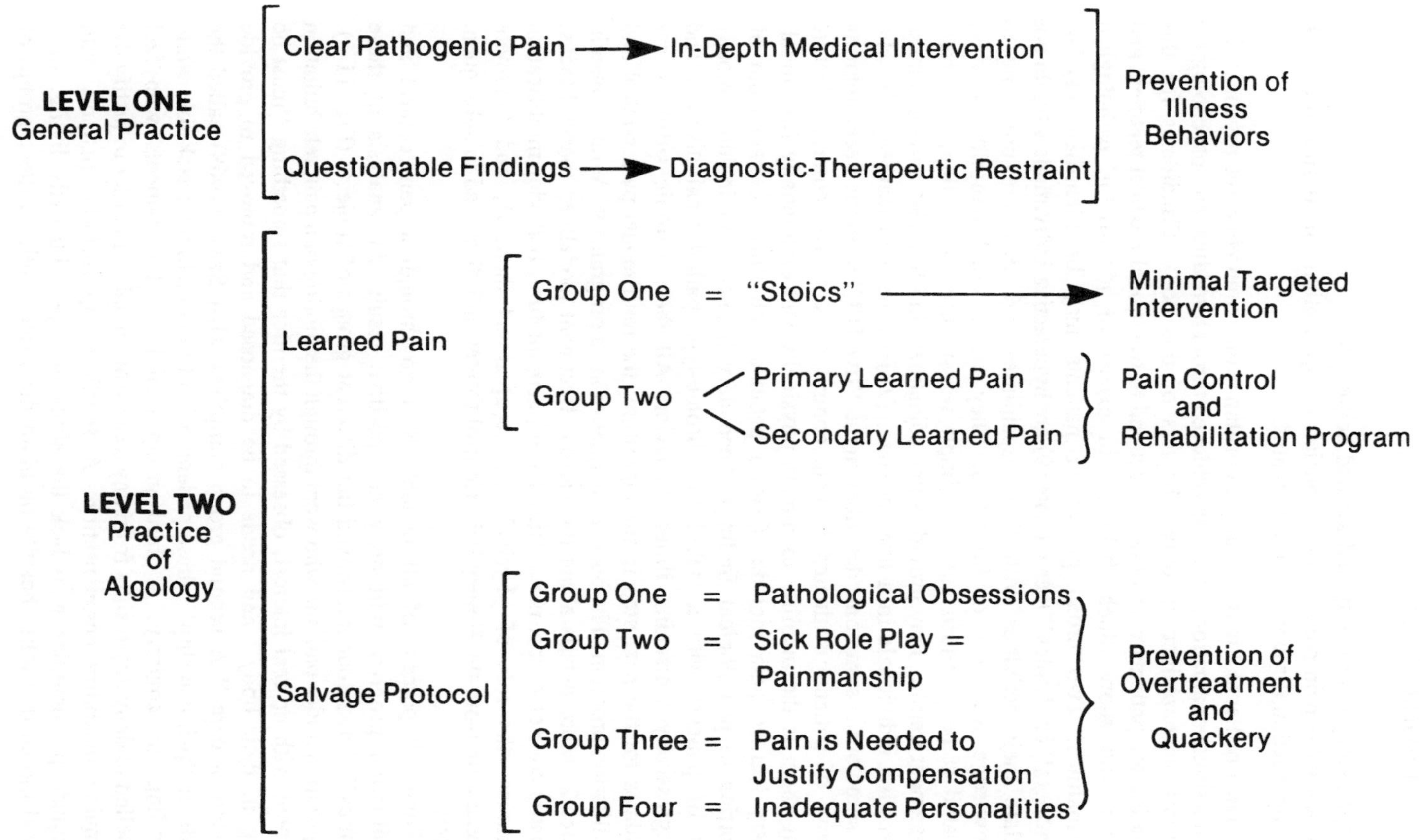

FIG. 11-2. Groups of subjects analyzed

4. Dependency—passivity and learned helplessness
5. Disability—pain-contingent financial compensation or desire for such compensation through disability claims.

Step 1 of Level 2 in the Emory algorithm is the comprehensive psychosocial and functional evaluation, which is achieved through medical and psychological teamwork as explained in other chapters of this book. Candidates for this evaluation are patients who failed to respond to traditional medical teatment and patients who show illness behavior in excess of identifiable pathological abnormalities. Two broad groups of patients may be identified: (1) The "overdoers" or "stoics" (see Chapter 9) are hyperactive individuals who do not correlate their activities with their capabilities and often are unwilling to acknowledge weakness or limitation. They are a small minority of those evaluated at pain control centers. Simple reassurance, counseling, and stress management training may provide some adjustment in life-styles and keep these hyperactive individuals in a healthy state. (2) Patients with learned pain who show some of the symptoms described in the "five D's" form the overwhelming majority of patients evaluated in pain control centers. The common feature among them is the inability to remain physically and emotionally functional. Primary learned pain includes Class I patients with illness behavior out of proportion to pathological findings. Secondary learned pain includes mostly Class III patients with a stabilized, chronic-type pathological disorder and a progressively worsening illness behavior. All these chronic sufferers are candidates for the next step in the algorithm: the multimodal pain control and rehabilitation program. The basic principles of such programs were mentioned in Chapter 2. More details about the various treatment modalities (nerve blocks, transcutaneous electrical nerve stimulation, acupuncture, behavior modification techniques, the role of physical and occupational therapy), and treatment outcome data from the Emory Pain Control Center, are discussed in subsequent chapters.

Some 30 percent of all patients who go through a pain control and rehabilitation program will deny any positive result. An analysis of these "failures" shows four intermixed but different groups of subjects (Fig. 11-2). One group includes patients who went through the motion of a pain rehabilitation treatment with no real interest, obsessed by the idea that something "must be wrong in their body" and needs to be diagnosed and removed to provide "permanent cure." A second group comprises what Szasz (1968) called the experts in "painmanship"; these patients wish to maintain their sick role while pretending the contrary. A third group includes a few patients who feel compelled to deny any results from any treatment modality in order to justify the continuing disability compensation. A fourth group includes patients with inadequate personalities who lack the skills to cope with daily living. In a medical milieu that relies heavily on biomedical interventions, these groups of

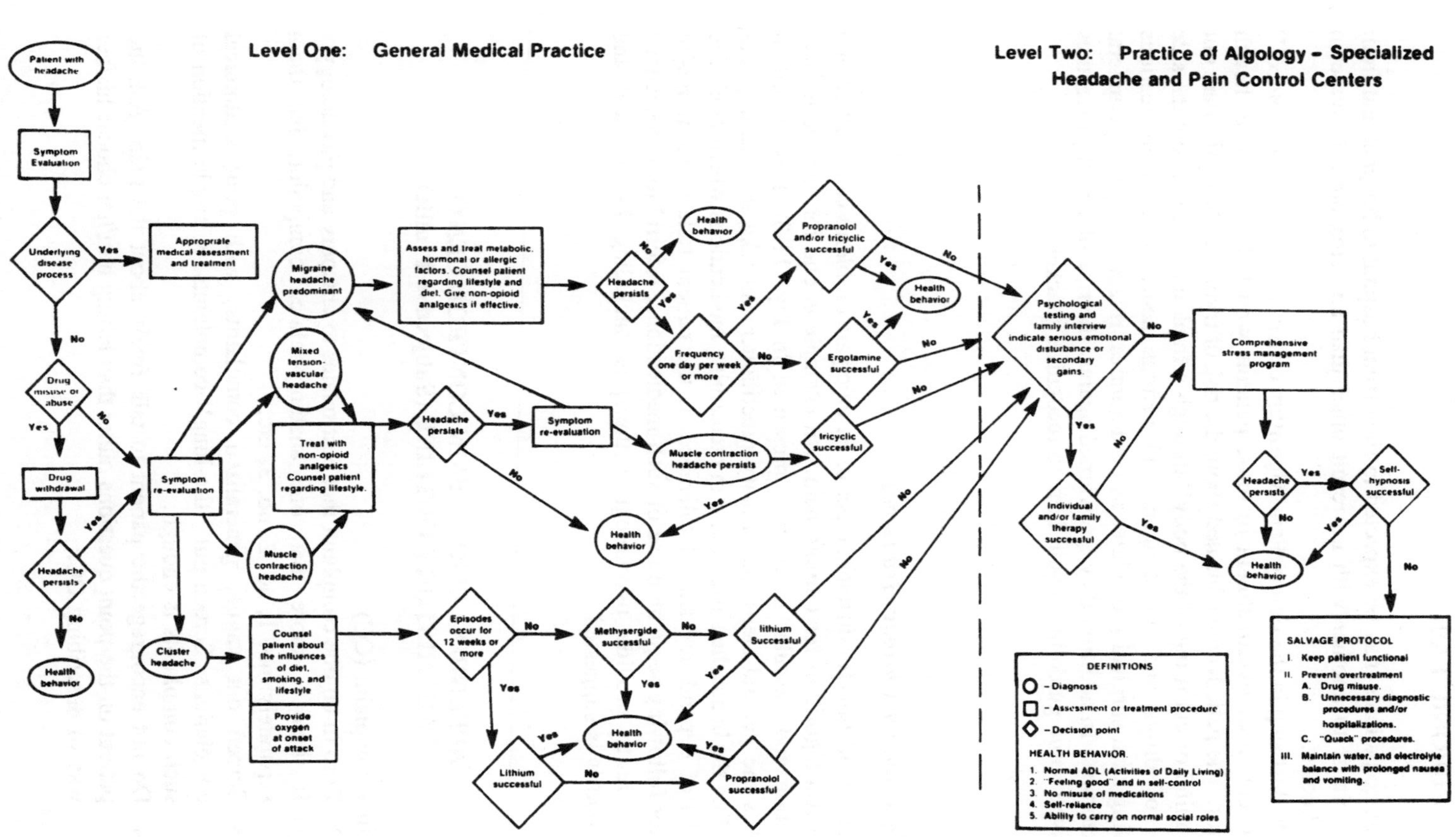

FIG. 11-3. An algorithm for decision-making in the assessment and treatment of chronic headache

unfortunate patients may be expected to float from hospital to hospital and from one specialist to another with no result other than an astronomic increase in medical costs.

The last step in the Emory Pain Algorithm consists of a "salvage protocol" for prevention of overtreatment in those patients who fail to return to health behavior. The patients are educated about the risk of trying to "drug the pain out of the mind or cut it out of the body" through a frank discussion about the side effects of drugs and the dangers and serious neurological complications following such surgical procedures as cordotomies, rhizotomies, and peripheral neurectomies. In addition they are warned against the risk of quack procedures and given some guidelines about how to recognize quackery.

An Algorithm for Chronic Headaches

Separate algorithms for different types of chronic pain problems can be fitted into the general algorithm for chronic pain. An example is one for chronic muscle contraction and vascular headaches, presented in Fig. 11-3. This algorithm describes the general steps the primary practitioner can take in assessing and counseling the headache sufferer and in prescribing medications which minimize the risks of dependency and of tolerance. If the patient fails to show health behavior following sequential use of such medications, referral to a specialized center able to provide psychological therapies including biofeedback and self-hypnosis is suggested.

APPENDIX. EMORY PAIN CONTROL CENTER PAIN HISTORY OUTLINE (Subjective Profile)

A. Chief complaint (CC)
   1. Zero in on one complaint that best relates to anatomy and physiology.
   2. If there is more than one anatomy-related complaint, list them separately: no. 1, no. 2, no. 3, etc.
   3. Screen out vague, generalized complaints, with poor anatomical correlations. Screen out "life-long" complaints. A single mention of such complaints is enough.
   4. Do not encourage the patient to talk freely about the pain. Ask the patient on-the-point questions rather than letting him/her choose his/her way of describing CC.

B. Onset

1. Establish the date of onset of CC, as you have identified it.
2. Document factors that precipitated CC, as the patient sees them. Establish relationship to job-connected injuries, and to accidents with a potential for, or in actual litigation.
3. Make a brief summary of what has been done medically for diagnosis and treatment of CC per patient's report and referring physician's notes.
4. Document dramatization of description of onset factors if any.

C. Pain description

1. Make patient choose between common-language bipolar verbal descriptors of pain: sharp–dull, deep–superficial, constant–intermittent, etc. Ask if there is a burning feeling.
2. Establish relationship between feelings and changes in activity levels, mostly with particular activities such as bending or lifting. Is pain increased by coughing, sneezing, straining etc.?
3. Ask for sleep and appetite disturbances. Does pain prevent patient from falling asleep or wake the patient up from sleep?
4. Establish relationship between pain intensity and changes in weather conditions.
5. Document dramatization, vagueness, and the imaginary in pain description (conditioned "pain language").
6. Watch facial expressions and posture while the patient is describing the pain. Do facial expression, postural attitudes, and other general indicators match with patient's verbal description of pain?
7. On a scale of 0 – 100 (0 = no pain, 100 = greatest amount of pain patient has ever experienced), ask patient to indicate the intensity of the pain, as experienced over the last week before the present interview.

D. Pain medication

1. Check all drugs the patients has taken since the onset of CC.
2. Check all drugs patient is taking for pain. List doses, frequency of intake, modality (p.r.n. versus time schedule).
3. List habit-forming drugs separately.
4. List drug allergies.

E. Past surgical history

1. List in retrograde surgical and medical episodes that relate to CC particularly.
2. Document possible occasions in the past medical history for learning sick behaviors. Was surgery done for a clear-cut pathological cause, or was it an "exploratory" surgery, that is, surgery because of pain complaints? How did the patient respond to treatment? Did the patient return to productive activities or move from one illness to another?

F. Social Profile

1. Age? Sex?
2. Married, divorced, widowed, or single?
3. Family composition. How many children at home?
4. Grade of education.
5. Professional or vocational training. How many jobs in the past five years? Satisfaction and performance with each.
6. Present job, or date of last workday.
7. Present income, or income from last paycheck.
8. Is patient on any disability income? How much? Is patient receiving Social Security benefits? Medical or retirement benefits?
9. Is patient seeking any disability benefits? Is there an attorney involved? Is there any actual legal claim or suit pending? If out of work, is the patient willing to be helped to return to work?
10. Are social and recreational activities gratifying? Decreased because of pain? What kind of social–recreational activities does the patient like to participate in, is actually participating in, or would like to participate in if relieved of pain?
11. How about the patient's sex life? Is it gratifying? Is it decreased because of pain?
12. How much uptime (time spent with feet on the floor) daily?
13. Any loss (economic, death, etc). in the family at or around the onset of CC?
14. Any change in environment (moves, etc.) at or around onset of CC?
15. How does patient see him/herself today as compared with one year ago? Happy? Depressed? Scared?
16. Effect of pain on family/social life.
17. Family attitude and behavior toward pain.

REFERENCES

Florence, D.W. 1979. Diary of work-related disability. *Legal Aspects Med. Pract.* Aug.

Szasz, T.S. 1968. The psychology of persistent pain: A portrait of the "Homo Dolorosus." in *Pain*, E. Soulairac (Ed.). New York: Academic Press.

12

Drugs and Pain: Use and Misuse

STEVEN F. BRENA

Scientific knowledge of the pharmacology of drugs is not always applied in the clinical use of drugs for pain where empiricism and misconception persist. Common pitfalls in drug medication for pain are briefly discussed. Various classes of drugs presently available for patients in pain are described with reference to their correct use, side effects, and misuse, as documented through the daily experience at the Emory Pain Control Center. Detoxification programs are described and a guideline for the use of drugs in chronic pain states is proposed.

The use of drugs to relieve various human ailments is one of the oldest forms of medical practice. The code of Hammurabi and several papyri of ancient Egypt refer to many drugs, such as opium, belladonna, hyosciamus, and hellebore. The writings of later famous physicians such as Dioscorides, Pliny the Elder, Galen, and Avicenna contain numerous prescriptions of herbs and drugs.

For centuries drugs were prescribed empirically with little knowledge of their actual mode of action and correct dosage. For instance, during the Middle Ages and up to the first three decades of the 19th century, a "spongia soporifera" (a somniferant sponge) was commonly used to induce sleep during amputation. Such a device was nothing more than a common sea sponge saturated with a mixture of opium, hyoscine, and mandragora juices. More than once the use of the soporific sponge must have progressed from sleep to death, since historians have recorded many examples of amputations performed without any analgesia in patients who probably feared death from the sponge more than they feared the agony of surgical pain (Brena, 1978).

Scientific knowledge on the pharmacology of drugs has greatly increased over the last four decades of the 20th century, sometimes with astonishing results. For example, the search for the mode of action of the opiates has led to the development of the new peptide neurophysiology of nociception, which is casting a new light on the nature of pain itself. Yet in clinical practice, a great deal of empiricism in the use of analgesic drugs and misconceptions about pain relief persist. There are many reasons for the pitfalls in drug medication for pain.

First, the assessment of analgesic drugs includes tests on both animal and human subjects. Animal tests may be valid for the species to which the animal belongs, but may not be valid for humans. For instance, analgesics of the salicylate type are usually ineffective in laboratory animals except in doses close to the LD-50 level. On the other hand, many drugs with proven analgesic effects on animals are not effective in humans. Clinical studies also are difficult because of the large number of factors that may influence outcome, such as dosage levels, patient selection, choice of controls, bias and placebo effects, and the impossibility of measuring objectively the subjective pain intensity.

Second, there is confusion about definitions of terms. The World Health Organization has defined addiction as "a behavior pattern of overwhelming involvement with obtaining and using a drug." In this definition addiction is a form of "drug abuse," defined as the use of any drug in a manner that elicits social disapproval. Both addiction and drug abuse refer to voluntary behaviors, and should not be confused with drug tolerance (decreased effectiveness of a given dosage after repeated doses) and physical dependence (withdrawal symptoms when a drug is discontinued), which refer to pharmacological effects. Whenever a prescription is given on a "prn for pain" basis, a medical–social approval for drug usage is granted; in fact the patient is given permission to request and obtain a drug "for pain," whether he/she really needs analgesic protection or not. Following p.r.n. prescriptions for pain in emotionally unstable patients, a conditioned pain-and-drug-seeking behavior, which is not related to actual nociception, is likely to develop quickly. The drug abuse is made socially acceptable through the legitimacy of physicians' prescriptions "for pain."

Third, many physicians are afraid of creating addiction to one particular drug, and choose to prescribe many different drugs for the same patients, at lower than optimal doses. In doing so they may unknowingly actually put the patient on the road to multiple-drug addiction, as cross-tolerance builds up.

Finally, consciously or not, the practicing physician will treat patients not only according to medical knowledge, but also in ways that will reflect his/her own personality, experience, and philosophy of life. For instance, a physician who habitually relies on self-control to deal with physical and emotional problems is less likely to prescribe drugs liberally, to the point of inadvertently denying adequate analgesia protection to patients with clear pathological nociception.

In common medical practice, various classes of drugs are available for patients in pain.

CENTRALLY ACTING ANALGESICS

Centrally acting analgesics include (1) opiates—the purified alkaloids of opium, such as morphine and codeine and their semisynthetic derivatives, such as

Dilaudid, Nubain, and oxycodone (in Percodan); (2) opioids—various synthetic compounds with morphine-like effects such as Demerol, Stadol, Nisentil, methadone, propoxyphene, and several others; and (3) a benzomorphan derivative, pentazocine (Talwin), with mixed agonist–antagonist effects with morphine.

The central analgesic drugs probably act as exogenous agonists of the endorphin-like endogenous regulation systems of pain perception. All opiates and opioids display cross-tolerance effects. The most commonly prescribed central analgesics in patients seen at the Emory Pain Control Center are codeine, propoxyphene, and oxycodone (Percodan), all of which have mild analgesic effects, approximately equivalent to acetaminophen in comparable doses (Moertel et al., 1972). All the central-acting oral analgesics have an additive effect with either aspirin or acetaminophen. More questionable is the additive effects of phenothiazines. For instance, promethazine (Phenergan) is frequently associated with the prescription of central analgesics, despite fairly conclusive evidence that it actually is an antianalgesic. (Halpern & Bonica, 1979). On the other hand, chlorpromazine (Thorazine) and promazine (Sparine) appear to have analgesic properties (Halpern & Bonica, 1979). Their strong sedative effects may be useful when the patient is hospitalized, but become a dangerous liability in the ambulatory patient. Alone or with other drugs in mixed analgesic combinations, the central analgesics can be used effectively in the management of pathogenic pain over short periods of time, in the nonambulatory patient. Actually, in the hospitalized patient, too often opiates are underprescribed because of fear of depression of the central nervous system. For instance, most of the opiates have an average duration of action that ranges between two and four hours, and yet the standard prescription for central analgesics is "q.4 h.," which needlessly exposes the patient to unnecessary discomfort as the blood level of the drug is at its lowest point at the end of the fourth hour, before the next dose is given.

Adverse reactions of central analgesics are well known and include respiratory depression, nausea, vomiting, constipation, cardiovascular effects, spasm of biliary and urinary tracts, and eventually an increase in spinal fluid pressure. Several mental processes are also impaired, with drowsiness, decrease in alertness and efficiency, clouding of the sensorium, and inability to think and concentrate clearly. Seizures may occur following intake of large doses of meperidine (Demerol). Adverse reactions may become serious health problems in the ambulatory chronic pain patient who is given prescriptions of central analgesic drugs over long periods of time, and needs progressively larger doses as tolerance develops. Constipation is a common complaint among chronic pain patients, resulting in dependency on laxatives. The constipation is corrected when the analgesics are discontinued. Inability to think clearly and to perform efficiently in common activities of daily living is another frequent complaint of chronic sufferers, who become needlessly frightened that they may have serious brain disease; in addition, the high drug usage confirms them strongly in the sick role and makes them poor candidates for pain rehabilitation. As the mental processes are cleared following elimination of the offending drugs, their attitude often changes dramatically; they become optimistic and comply enthusiastically with subsequent rehabilitation.

An unquestionable example of drug misuse, not infrequently documented in our own experience, is the concomitant use of an opiate and of pentazocine, which is an opiate antagonist. The end result is a potentiation of adverse reactions of both drugs with little analgesic effect in an emotionally drained patient.

PERIPHERALLY ACTING ANALGESICS

The peripherally acting analgesics include aspirin, acetaminophen (Tylenol), and the newer nonsteroidal anti-inflammatory agents, such as ibuprofen (Motrin), naproxen (Naprosyn), sulindac (Clinoril), and phenylbutazone (Butazolidin). Several studies (Bloomfield. et al., 1974, 1976, 1977) have shown that aspirin, whose first use dates back to 1899, is still one of the best analgesic drugs in the ambulatory patient, especially when the painful state is associated with acute and semiacute inflammatory processes. Aspirin and other salicylates have been shown to inhibit the synthesis of prostaglandins, which are involved in complex biochemical interreactions with various neurotransmitters of the still poorly understood pain-modulating system.

Adverse reactions to aspirin are well known, and include gastrointestinal symptoms, gastric distress, changes in prothrombin time and platelet aggregation, which affect blood coagulation, and symptoms of neurotoxicity, such as tinnitus, dizziness, and confusion.

The single most dangerous factor associated with aspirin is its easy availability as a drug sold without medical prescription. Many chronic pain patients develop compulsive needs to gulp down pills; they buy various over-the-counter preparations with different trade-names, but all containing aspirin in various dosages. Unknown to them, and often to their physicians, they develop symptoms of gastric distress and neurotoxicity, become frightened, and as a result increase their illness behaviors. The damage is compounded when aspirin is associated with phenacetin and caffeine in the numerous so-called APC preparations. Several patients at the Emory Pain Control Center have developed unexplained renal and urinary tract malfunctions (''analgesic nephropathy''), whose roots may be traced to compulsive and prolonged use of APC preparations. Even more dangerous are the APC compounds containing an opiate; as tolerance to the opiate develops, larger doses of the compound drug are taken, thus combining the adverse reactions of aspirin, phenacetin and the opiates upon the gastrointestinal, hepatic, and urinary systems.

An excellent peripheral analgesic drug is acetaminophen, with a rate of efficiency slightly inferior to that of aspirin, but with no anti-inflammatory effect. The only serious complication associated with gross overdose of acetaminophen is hepatic damage. Though cases of death from hepatic necrosis have been reported, no hepatic damage has been observed at the Emory Pain Control Center in thousands of patients compulsively misusing acetaminophen.

The newer nonsteroidal anti-inflammatory peripheral analgesics are marketed as specific antiarthritic agents; they almost duplicate the effects of aspirin, with fewer but similar adverse reactions. No serious misuse of these anti-inflammatory drugs has yet been observed in chronic pain patients, and no complication has been documented from these drugs at the Emory Pain Control Center.

A particular analgesic drug worth mentioning here is carbamazepine (Tegretol), a tricyclic compound chemically related to imipramine. The drug is the agent of first choice for the treatment of tic douloureux of the trigeminal and glossopharyngeal nerves, either alone or in concomitant use with diphenylhydantoin (Dilantin) (Loeser, 1977). Carbamazepine has also been reported useful in the treatment of various denervation syndromes affecting the central nervous system, such as causalgia, post-herpetic neuralgia, diabetic neuropathy (Davis et al., 1977), phantom limb pain, and pain following spinal cord injuries (Loeser, 1975).

The incidence of multiple and serious adverse reactions to carbamazepine is high and the drug should be used with caution and under continuous medical supervision. Probably because of such restrictions, no cases of carbamazepine misuse have been observed at the Emory Pain Control Center.

SEDATIVES AND ANTIANXIETY AGENTS

The sedatives and antianxiety agents comprise a variety of chemicals, which share in common the capability of inducing sedation and sleep through depression of the central nervous system. They include barbiturates, benzodiazepines, meprobamate, hydroxyzine, bromides, quaalude, chloral derivatives, glutethimide, and alcohol. Since the advent of the benzodiazepines, barbiturates and other sedatives are used less frequently for insomnia and daytime sedation. Through skillful advertising within the medical media, the benzodiazepines, especially diazepam (Valium), have become the most overprescribed drugs in the United States. Sedatives and so-called "tranquilizers" have no proven analgesic effect, and yet they are among the drugs most often prescribed for chronic pain patients.

Adverse reactions include drowsiness and impairment of mental alertness, physical coordination, and judgment. With higher doses, ataxia, feelings of chronic fatigue, sexual impotence and frigidity, gastrointestinal distress, skin rashes, and blood dyscrasias have been reported. Pharmacodynamic tolerance develops quickly with the use of most sedatives and antianxiety agents. Moreover, barbiturates, glutethimide, and chloral hydrate induce hepatic microsomal enzymes, which may increase the rate of hepatic metabolism of many drugs that may be used at the same time, such as coumarin and tricyclic antidepressants.

Benzodiazepines and other sedatives often are prescribed in combination with central and peripheral analgesics. Controlled studies of the effectiveness of such mixtures have given conflicting results; thus, with very few exceptions, there is little reason for using them in preference to a single agent. In the experience at the Emory Pain Control Center, one of the most common offenders in terms of adverse reactions and physical dependence is Fiorinal, a mixture of APC and a barbiturate, butalbital (50 mg), with or without codeine. Fiorinal has been advertised as a drug of choice for muscle-contraction headaches. Because many such tension syndromes are intermittent with variable frequency, many patients given a p.r.n. prescription of Fiorinal have habitually taken it continuously in the false belief that it will prevent onset of future headache episodes. As tolerance to the barbiturates and/or codeine develops, the doses are increased, signs of APC overdosage appear, and the patient becomes emotionally drained and incapacitated. Following detoxification and biofeedback training, most of these patients return to healthy life patterns with fewer intermittent headaches.

The misuse of antianxiety agents and sedatives is a serious health problem, leading to a variety of disabling illness behaviors far in excess of any detectable pathological or emotional problem. The drug history preceding injuries or accidents often reveals several common scenarios: the ambulatory working individual who had prescriptions for Valium, Librium, Dalmane, etc., "p.r.n. for sleep at bedtime," and actually had been taking these pills several times day and night; the patient out of work "because of pain," who is actually dysfunctional because of the adverse reactions to unnecessary prescriptions of sedatives and "tranquilizers"; the patient frightened into total inactivity by the obsession of having a deadly disease, following the drug-induced alteration of mental activity. Many of these iatrogenic sufferers do show evidence of maladjusted personalities on Minnesota Multiphasic Personality Inventory testing, with histories of poor existential coping with the stresses of daily living; many express feelings of insecurity through maladaptive pain and illness behaviors. Their feelings of insecurity and inadequacy, however, are compounded by the drug-induced mental confusion. When detoxified and trained to improve their coping skills through rehabilitation programs, most of them return to more normal life-styles.

MUSCLE RELAXANTS AND ANTIDEPRESSANTS

Muscle spasm is one of the most common complaints in patients displaying maladaptive illness behaviors. A number of drugs, chemically related to the antianxiety agents, are marketed as "central muscle relaxants": carisoprodol (Soma), methocarbamol (Robaxin), orphenadrine (Norflex), cyclobenzaprine (Flexeril), which is a tryciclic compound, and a few others. These drugs are claimed to be useful in cases of fibrositis, arthritis, and bursitis. All of these drugs produce depression in neuronal activity affecting muscle stretch reflexes. They also produce mild sedation; the subjective pain relief may be due both to mild sedation and to the depressed central neuronal activity. No adverse reaction or physical dependence has been observed in patients taking muscle relaxant drugs at the Emory Pain Control Center.

The only true peripheral muscle relaxant is dantrolene (Dantrium), which is beneficial in the treatment of spasticity, and does not significantly affect mental alertness and coordination.

Depression has been mentioned throughout this book as one of the common symptoms associated with chronic pain states; it is usually expressed through feelings of helplessness, sleeplessness, inactivity, and social withdrawal. It stands to reason that any drug—or other nonchemical treatment modality—capable of correcting these symptoms could alter the suffering experience. Among the antidepressant agents, the tricyclic compounds, especially doxepin (Sinequan) and amitriptyline (Elavil), have gained acceptance and are frequently prescribed for chronic pain patients.

Actually none of these drugs has any proven analgesic effects in acute pain; however, the feelings of increased physical fitness and the improved mental alertness, appetite, and sleep patterns often serve to reduce morbid preoccupation and help promote increase in activity and improved social adjustment.

Among the multiple adverse reactions induced by the tricyclic compounds, the most commonly observed are mild anticholinergic and alpha-adrenergic blocking activities (dryness of the mouth, blurred vision, constipation, urinary retention, and diaphoresis). Sedation and, paradoxically, insomnia may also occur. Seizures have been reported. Physical dependency may develop and withdrawal symptoms have been observed after these drugs have been abruptly discontinued.

Several headache clinics in the United States have suggested the use of tricyclic antidepressants as drugs of first choice for muscle-tension headaches (Kudrow, 1980; Chapman & Brena, 1980). Alone, or in combination with Tegretol and Dilantin, the tricyclic compounds also have been reported useful in the treatment of post-herpetic and other neuralgias (Davis et al., 1977; Crue et al., 1975).

DETOXIFICATION PROGRAMS

Most chronic pain patients do not like to take drugs. They dimly realize that drugs are useless in relieving their suffering, but continue to take them compulsively, short of alternatives. At the Emory Pain Control Center, all patients accepted for evaluation and treatment are asked to attend a taped one-hour informative lecture, during which the adverse reactions of drugs for pain are explained, along with other aspects of chronic pain syndromes (the "five D's"). Following the lecture many patients demonstrate willingness to discontinue drug medication, and ask for instructions and alternatives. When physical dependence is not a problem, patients are instructed to discontinue medication gradually at home with frequent follow-ups at the Center, and are given training in progressive relaxation exercises to deal with feelings of anxiety, muscle spasms, and difficulties in sleeping. If physical dependence is suspected, patients are hospitalized for drug detoxification. Patients who are taking opiates are able to discontinue their medication in a relatively short time and with little discomfort. Those taking benzodiazepines, however, usually go through longer periods of relative discomfort, because of the long plasma half-lives (up to eight days) of these drugs. The few patients taking glutethimide show the longest period of discomfort, probably because of the well-known activity of a potent active metabolite of the drug.

Phase I

Patients are instructed to bring with them all drugs they habitually take at home and turn them over to the ward nurse on admission. During the first 24 hours after admission, a baseline drug profile is taken. The patient is placed in a closed environment and given whatever drugs he/she requests on a p.r.n. basis. A registered nurse administers the drugs and keeps records. After 24 hours a drug profile listing the type and quantity of drugs and intake patterns for each patient can be constructed. All p.r.n. orders for opiates, sedatives, and antianxiety agents are discontinued at the end of Phase I.

Phase II

Use of opiates is switched to equivalent doses of methadone; sedatives and antianxiety agents are switched to phenobarbital equivalents; pentazocine is withdrawn independently.

Methadone and phenobarbital are given in a liquid vehicle on an exact-time contingency. After a switchover period of 24 hours and stabilization, methadone doses are decreased by 20 percent daily; phenobarbital doses are decreased by 10 percent each day; pentazocine is usually discontinued within three days independently of predetoxification levels. Supportive therapy, mostly recreational therapy, is recommended.

Spouses and other close relatives are educated through group counseling sessions about the dangers of drug misuse and the learning factors associated with compulsive drug dependency. Patients are seen regularly and are reassured about withdrawal symptoms.

Patients detoxified from drug misuse usually do not relapse. Long-term changes in drug use are presented in Chapter 14.

GUIDELINES FOR USE OF DRUGS IN CHRONIC PAIN STATES

1. The use of any sedative or antianxiety agent in the functional pain patient is a potential misuse.
2. The use of opiates should be limited to nonambulatory patients in cases of clear pathogenic pain, from a progressive and invasive disease process. When the decision to use opiates is made, the drug must be given in doses high enough to provide effective analgesia.
3. In cases of chronic pain associated with a nonprogressive, noninvasive pathological process of long duration, the drug of first choice is probably a tricyclic antidepressant, not a central nervous system depressant agent. If a rheumatic-type inflammatory process is documented, a nonsteroidal anti-inflammatory drug may be added. Activities rather than inactivity should be promoted to avoid fostering sick roles in chronic sufferers.
4. No drug for chronic pain should be prescribed on a p.r.n. basis. Time-contingent prescriptions are less likely to lead to drug misuse through conditioning. Compulsive demands from the patient should be resisted and drugs never should be prescribed without proper assessment and follow-up.
5. Patients should be educated and informed. If given proper information about drug reactions, most of them will voluntarily limit drug intake and exercise self-control to maintain function and avoid misuse.
6. Alternative treatment modalities should be provided. Many patients requesting drugs for sleep and muscle spasms will report no further need for the drugs after they have successfully learned relaxation skills. Taped audiovisual teaching of such exercises will not tax the professional time of the busy practitioner.

REFERENCES

Bloomfield, S.S., Barden, T.P., and Mitchell, J. 1974. Comparative efficacy of ibuprofen and aspirin in episiotomy pain. *Clin. Pharmacol. Therap.* 15:565–570.

Bloomfield, S.S., Barden, T.P., and Mitchell, J. 1976. Aspirin and codeine in two postpartum pain models. *Clin. Pharmacol. Therap.* 20:499–503.

Bloomfield, S.S., Barden, T.P., and Mitchell, J. 1977. Naproxen, aspirin and codeine in postpartum uterine pain. *Clin. Pharmacol. Therap.* 21:414–421.

Brena, S.F., 1978. Pain and drug misuse. In *Chronic Pain: America's Hidden Epidemic*. New York: Atheneum.

Chapman, S.L., and Brena, S.F. 1980. An algorithm for decision making in patients with headache. Presented at Second Annual Meeting, American Pain Society, New York, Sept.

Crue, B.L., Todd, E.M., and Maline, D.B.M. 1975. Post-herpetic neuralgia—Conservative treatment regimen. In *Pain: Research and Treatment*, B.L. Crue (Ed.). New York: Academic Press.

Davis, J.L., Gerich, J.E., and Schultz, T.A. 1977. Peripheral diabetic neuropathy treated with amitriptyline and fluphenothiazine. *JAMA* 238:2291–2292.

Halpern, L.M., and Bonica, J.J. 1979. Analgesics. In *Drugs of Choice*, W. Modell. (Ed.). St. Louis: C.V. Mosby.

Kudrow, L. 1980. Analgesics and headache. *Postgrad. Med. Commun.* 51–63.

Loeser, J.D. 1975. Central pains. *Clin. Med.* 82:24–25.

Loeser, J.D. 1977. Management of tic douloureux. *Pain* 3:155–162.

Moertel, C.G., Ahmann, D.L., Taylor, W.F., and Schwartau, N. 1972. *N. Engl. J. Med.* 15:813–815.

13

Milieu Psychotherapy

RICHARD H. MORSE

All psychotherapy with chronic pain must be diverted toward replacing pain-related behavior with normal activity. This goal can be achieved through careful structuring of the environment or "milieu" with a program of structured activities and careful handling of patients' regressions and crises. Family therapy, group therapy, and sexual counseling are important components of pain management that can be performed with some training and guidance by the general practitioner. Although individual psychotherapy with the chronic pain patient requires considerable experience and training, the general practitioner can provide important guidance and supportive therapy.

GENERAL PRINCIPLES

Psychotherapy in the form of a one-to-one relationship of the therapist to the patient is by no means the most common modality of emotional treatment for the chronic pain patient. When used it is usually combined with other therapies: the use of the *milieu* (environment) itself in the form of a therapeutic community, group psychotherapy, conjoint family therapy, and specialized sessions such as sexual counseling.

General Goals of Chronic Pain Treatment

Regardless of whether we employ a surgical, medical, or emotional approach to the chronic pain patient, the guiding treatment goal remains unchanged:

pain related behavior --------→normal activity
(replaced by)

When pain behavior is replaced by normal activity, the patient perceives the quality of life improved, as activity itself is one of the strongest antidepressant modalities both emotionally and physiologically. In addition activity is itself a powerful analgesic, possibly mediated through the effect of increased endorphin release during exercise. Seldom in chronic pain treatment can the patient become totally pain-free, a fact that must be exceedingly clear to the therapist, the patient, and the family. The situation is very similar to alcoholic treatment in this respect; we strive for an active patient with diminished pain, who can cope with relapses early on, just as we strive for a "dry" or abstinent alcoholic who may never lose the identity with the drinking problem.

Review of the "Disease of D's"

Any psychotherapeutic approach must overcome the basic life-style into which the chronic pain patient and family have fallen. This life-style is represented by the D's as follows:

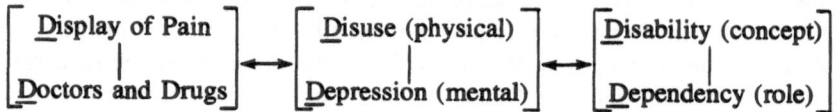

Display of Pain	↔	Disuse (physical)	↔	Disability (concept)
Doctors and Drugs		Depression (mental)		Dependency (role)

Disability represents a self-concept, however it has been taught or acquired; indeed we often see severely impaired patients such as quadriplegics who return to work. Dependency, however, is a social role, often involving the family and the medical caretakers. A psychotherapeutic approach inevitably aims at these two areas, regardless of modality chosen.

Splitting and Alexithymia

Chronic pain patients, although not appearing overtly regressed or psychotic, "split" the images through which they see others into "good" and "bad" stereotypes, in total disregard for reality. This splitting is protective psychologically, meant to guard loved persons or aspects of the self from rage (Mahler, 1979). Furthermore chronic pain patients have great difficulty in perceiving that they are even experiencing a negative emotion (such as anger, guilt, or anxiety), and have much difficulty in differentiating emotions. The inability to read one's emotions is called "alexithymia," excellently discussed by Nemiah (1978). The psychotherapist must be continually sensitive to and accepting of these pathological features of the patient and must be gentle enough to avoid the great pitfall of exposing the patient to his/her strong negative emotions without defenses.

The Pain Game

The transactions of the chronic pain patient fit the following adapted model of "gamesmanship" so brilliantly described by Berne (1964).

The "Pain Game"

Basic assumptions:
1. The pain belongs to the doctor (not the patient).
2. The doctor can "take it back" with drugs, or surgery.

The "con" (false reward/punishment system):
1. If the doctor succeeds, then the doctor is "believed."
2. If the doctor fails, then the doctor must feel guilty and will be either "hated" or "forgiven" by the patient.

The "script":
1. For the doctor: "fail and be guilty" (patient will guide doctor)
2. For the patient: "hurt"

When this game is played out according to these rules, the results are relapses, overmedication, polysurgery (beyond the indicated), and excessive referrals. Breaking the Pain Game is basically simple in concept, and in no way damages the dignity of the doctor or patient. It is based on two basic assumptions: (1) the pain belongs to the patient; and (2) the doctor is part of a team to help the patient cope.

The simplicity of these new assumptions is deceptive, because an experienced patient will almost inevitably undo the best efforts of the team members. Regardless of the modality of psychotherapy, these new assumptions or "contracts" must be maintained. Team members must be trained to empathize with the patient's unhappiness and difficulties, but refuse to assume the role of "curers." This role is often particularly difficult for physicians, but they usually are delighted with its effectiveness.

The Task

In summary the central task in chronic pain treatment, regardless of modality, is to: (1) convert pain-related behavior into normal activity, (2) counteract the "D's"; (3) cause the patient to assume "problem ownership" of illness; and (4) avoid pitfalls of primitive splitting, alexithymia, and self-demoralization in the patient.

MILIEU THERAPY: THERAPEUTIC COMMUNITY AND STRUCTURED PROGRAM

The central tasks outlined can be accomplished if we look to the treatment environment or "milieu" as a source of skill, authority, and support; it is, after all, within the environments of family, school, and the outside world that both sick and well emotions and behaviors are created or undone. This form of treatment allows the therapist and patient to relate to each other amid the molding, reshaping forces of a group, and allows the primary physician to stand back and assume medical direction for treatment while extricating him/herself from the misplaced dependency of the patient. Pain patients readily accept the presence of other pain patients, but typically make self-defeating attempts to re-create their chronic pain environment instead of learning new skills and behaviors. Because they are working as a team, staff members can provide each other with support, ventilation, and strategy to counteract these attempts. This task would be impossible in the medical office.

Much of the impact of the milieu stems from its structure:

1. The *location* of the program is usually in a separate facility or section. Proximity of pain patients to other patients is workable only if there is complete understanding of the pain patients' uniqueness.
2. The physical setting and design of the program are much like a residential school, avoiding the isolation and passive support provided by either the acute hospital or home.
3. The *daily living activities* of the program resemble normal life, being neither too undertaxing, nor too overtaxing. Patients may cook and serve themselves or each other at meals, everybody wears ordinary clothes, laundry and supplies are available, and patients have access to "out trips" for entertainment, shopping, etc., with staff as required.
4. Thorough *information* is provided and *contracts* are formulated and signed with family and staff during the initial staff hours. Included are agreements to attend activities and family sessions, delegate medication to the staff, etc.
5. *Transition* to and from the *program and home* is formalized with gradually increasing opportunities for the patient to be home. Usually a three-to-six-week inpatient phase is followed by an outpatient program after careful contracts and specific plans for outpatient activities are made.
6. *Group identification* and *staff advocacy* are employed; beginning patients support each other as they enter the program and are taught by the more advanced patients. By the end of the program, most patients will have developed close relationships with selected staff and patients. Each patient has a non-physician staff coordinator or advocate to help to structure the patient's program, communicate with the family, and intentionally wean the patient from seeing the physician as the source of all skills.
7. A program of *structured activities* is the backbone of any program. The patient's day revolves around activities rather than the chronic pain problem. Each attempt by the patient to reduce the program to sole reliance on the physician is greeted with empathy but a strong imperative and encouragement

to "do the program," so as to achieve the success modeled by the more advanced patients. The following is a typical day's activities, each of which counteracts the "disease of D's":

Arising and bed-making (often a rare event at home)
Morning medication (by the nurse's watch, few p.r.n.'s)
Breakfast (together and with staff)
Movement therapy (modified dance, therapies for gait, posture, and expression)
Group therapy (with staff, and family on visiting days)
Lunch (with staff)
"Doctors' rounds" (never in patient's room)
Occupational/vocational therapy (includes out-trips)
Relaxation training (musculoskeletal, breathing, etc.)
Dinner (together or outside with family, not at home)
Recreation and socialization

8. Other *complementary treatments* are provided as needed, including medical consultations, detoxification "by the clock" from all sedative narcotic substances, medication through antidepressants, anti-inflammatory, and nonnarcotic muscle-relaxant drugs, and family, couple, and sexual counseling.

The conduct of such a structured program is intended, if it is truly functional, to provoke two central events: the patients' attempts at *regression* to their dysfunctional patterns and *crises*. Though the uninitiated therapist may see these events as the undoing of a program, the experienced team sees them as heralding the patients' engagement in treatment and providing the basic material for therapy. Indeed, it is mostly during regressed states that learning occurs. This therapeutic regression follows a predictable course during milieu treatment: during the first days the patient is passive, angry, confused, or brave, but soon becomes highly child-like and creates a miniature family constellation among significant staff members. In structuring a "normal" activity pattern, the program allows transient dependency, limit setting, and gradual reentry into activity.

The emotional or pain "crises" occur throughout all phases of the program, suddenly or gradually, and usually represent brief intense regression or frank resistance to the "well role." To handle the crises, basic crisis intervention techniques suffice, centering on the immediate events precipitating the reaction, and allowing nonexplosive expression of emotion; great care must be taken to allow the patient to take control of the situation and to avoid being rescued by the treatment team.

Thus the role of the staff is to recognize regressions, crises, and other resistances, to avoid being overwhelmed by them, and to return to the basic goal of replacing pain behaviors with normal activities. Needless to say, a definite program of staff meetings is required to preserve the sanity and effectiveness of the team. Skill in milieu therapy requires literally years of experience for team leaders and members; however, a well-established team can train new recruits quickly to a point of basic competence and ability to handle amazingly diverse situations.

The intensive use of a specialized therapeutic community and structured program allows the greatest implementation of relearning opportunities as well as support for the necessary physical and emotional treatments. However, successful treatment with a more limited approach is possible if a primary physician works with a counsulting algologist and a pain team including a social worker, nurse, and delegate from occupational and physical therapy. The pain patients in a general or rehabilitation hospital can be detoxified and often placed on antidepressants, and can receive group, physical, and occupational therapy, participate in educational and family sessions, and share a community room. The treatment team should have training or experinece in an established pain unit elsewhere to ensure competence in treatment.

GROUP THERAPY

Group psychotherapy is the most common form of psychotherapy used in chronic pain treatment on an inpatient or outpatient level. Chapman (see Chapter 14) discusses the usefulness and role of group therapy in the general context of cognitive behavior modification. Briefly these uses include education in the theory and course of treatment, management of expectations, enhancement of cooperation, diminution of "aloneness," expression of negative, harmfully repressed affects, plus handing down of coping skills and hope from the more advanced to the newcomers.

Beyond these qualities a group has more general healing aspects, as enumerated by Slavson (1979): It helps to reduce resistance, to dilute and modify otherwise unmanageable transferences, to allow patients to observe themselves, and to provide a catalyst and forum for improved reality testing. Indeed, some initially threatening events, such as conflict between co-therapists, can have growth value. Yalom (1975) points out that observing the two therapists differentiate as individuals can strengthen the honesty and potency of the whole group, literally allowing it to spring into life.

In their interactions pain patients frequently take on the role of "help-rejecting complainers," who take pride in the insolubility of their problems and reject the help offered them. The presence of a group in which patients are free to complain often is therapeutic, even though it threatens the sanity of the therapists. Referring to the LAD schema of Chapter 5 (see Fig. 13-1), expression of a justified shared complaint removes guilt and denial, and thus allows the ventilation of anger that has culminated from latent depression and a sense of loss. Central to this process is the conversion of painful behavior to normal activity: unacceptable emotions, expressed as bodily pain, reach socially acceptable verbal levels.

With experience co-therapists will develop their own favorite ingenious ploys in group therapy. A therapist declaring his or her own helplessness in the face of the insatiable demands and demoralization of the patients often is greeted by a surge of self-assertiveness; "paradoxical intent," such as by suggesting the overrescue of a "helpless" patient, can create an intolerable position for the whole group, with a patient usually engaging in self-extrication; mention of a hidden external authority, for example the rumor that the director felt that an impossible group had been admitted, promotes group consolidation.

Chronic pain psychotherapy groups are unlike traditional groups. They cannot be categorized as being oriented toward task, process, transition, or support because the patients' dynamics tend to be arrested at a level often more primitive than that of neurotic or even psychotic patients, even though the pain patients may appear more stable.

Many private physicians and pain specialists regularly conduct their own group therapy. There is no better way to train for chronic pain group therapy than to work with an experienced therapist in an actual group, with complete anticipation that this experience will be substantially different from any other.

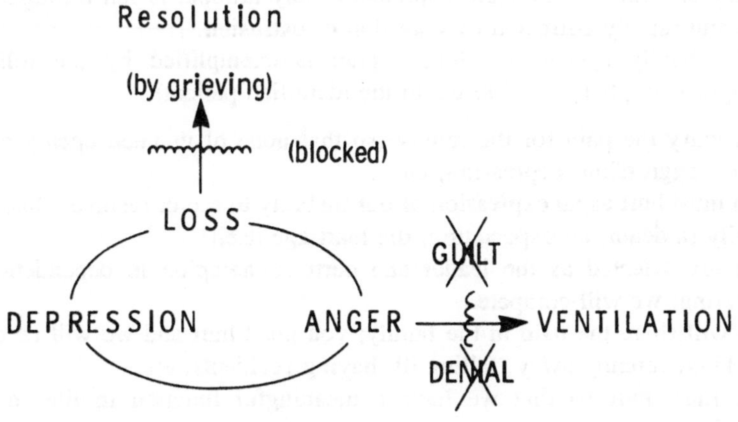

FIG. 13-1. LAD schema (see also Chapter 5)

FAMILY THERAPY

The strongest reinforcement of pain behavior and strongest resistance to adaptation will be found in the family network in which the patient has been selected for the long-term, sick, disabled, dependent, and hurting role. As indicated in Chapter 5, the patient and family mutually condition each other to maintain the painful *status quo*; in fact the patient customarily relapses upon the first therapeutic home visit. The widest swings in patient improvement or deterioration occur following communication with the family and direction of change depends on whether there has been adequate family involvement in the program.

Family intervention takes place throughout every phase of treatment. Even the initial interview and orientation should include as many family members as workable. From the outset a contract specifying the frequency and manner with which the family will participate must be reached, and usually signed. Families are expected to attend orientation meetings, social history intakes, and couples and family therapy sessions. Often family visits are "rewards" for completion of activity and the family will stand back during periods when the patient is attempting to use independent skills in overcoming crises.

The "systems theory" allows one to understand family interactions. This theory holds that all parts of the family are in contact with each other and that the family attempts to maintain a given equilibrium (whether healthy or "sick"). Any movement or stimulus inside or outside the family will be greeted by an energetic response, always directed at restoring the usual equilibrium. An intuitive model of this theory is the spider web: a nearly invisible, enormously strong but plastic structure, all points being held in place by strict structural geometry or "rule." The mere approach of any intruder is felt throughout the system and rapidly corrected by digestion or extrusion.

The family system in chronic pain is exemplified by the following pathological scripts ("you" refers to the identified patient).

1. You carry the pain for the family (so that none of us need openly express anger, aggression, depression, etc.).
2. You must hurt as an expression of our inability to see or resolve a loss in the family (a death, an expectation, the marriage itself).
3. You are selected as the leader and current champion in dependency and suffering; we will compete.
4. We will share the pain in the family; you must hurt and we will take turns drinking, running away, falling ill, having accidents, etc.
5. You must hurt so that we have a meaningful function in life, namely, rescuing.

Most of these unadaptive roles are meant to cover up unacceptable impulses or areas of intense vulnerability. A layering of defenses takes place in the family. The pain problem covers the familial anger and anxiety, the surface or harsh emotions; these in turn cover the deeper and more vulnerable feelings of helplessness, grief, etc. Often there is a conflict between needs in a family (i.e., to emancipate or individuate is to destroy the family and lose one's base of support or nurture). The more vulnerable feelings frequently relate to previous generations in the family, making it advantageous in therapy to have several generations present or to discuss scripts or "messages" from previous generations.

The therapeutic process involves progressing the family from the defensive and superficial harsher affects toward expression of the more vulnerable feeling states. Family myths or scripts are discussed and families can role-play new versus old behavioral patterns. Communications and assertiveness skills are taught and the family's basic competence is emphasized in training them to recognize and solve their problems independently. Many primary physicians have learned family therapy in brief programs offered in the community and excel in it.

SEXUAL COUNSELING

In the central goal of converting pain-related behavior to normal activity, the restoration of sexual activity is often overlooked but is of primary importance to the sense of independence and capacity of the chronic pain patient. The "D's" of depression, disuse, and disability predominate. Actually the experience of chronic pain need in no way itself interfere with sexual desire and relations, although marked interruption can arise from depression, drug effects, weakness, and orthopedic restriction, to which the patient must be taught to adapt. Though concerned with resuming sexual activity, the patient usually has not brought it up or has received evasive or inappropriate advice, such as to "resume things but take it easy." Eliciting a direct and supportive sexual history, preferably with the spouse or "significant other" person present, is usually accepted by the patient with both a feeling of comfort and of relief. The actual counseling may be conducted by anybody on the team who is comfortable and experienced in doing so, although an opposite-sex pair of co-therapists is ideal. The task is easier if the problem is inhibition of previously established sex lives, rather than prior dysfunction. Under ordinary circumstances, however, the sexual counseling of chronic pain patients is exceedingly simple, by no means requiring a full training in sexual therapies.

Though overlooking a physical or pharmacological cause of dysfunction in the initial history and physical examination is a major pitfall, overly elaborate focus on physical etiologies usually is unnecessary. A brief urogenital history, including inquiry regarding bladder and bowel sphincter function, especially urinary hesitancy, dribbling or incontinence, is helpful. Of male patients one should inquire regarding nocturnal or morning erection and presence of masturbatory erection and ejaculation; of female patients one should ask about pain on penetration, during defecation, etc. A brief neurological examination of sensory areas and of reflexes (ankle jerks, cremasteric, etc.) should be conducted with both sexes; an excellent measure is the combination of electrodiagnostic studies [electromyelograms (EMG), nerve conduction] plus cystometrogram (preferably including sphincter EMG). Diabetic imbalances and problems stemming from use of all narcotics and strongly anticholinergic drugs also should be corrected; psychotropic medications should be taken *after* intercourse. Detoxification from narcotics is much facilitated by explaining to the patient the possiblity of sexual recovery.

The sexual/emotional history is actually the beginning of therapy, since implicit in it is the interest of the physician, the suggestion that sexual function may be possible, and a basic but impactful permission-giving to "be sexual again." Consideration of the following questions is essential.

1. What changes have occurred sexually since the onset of illness? Frequency of intercourse is of minor importance compared with the mutual satisfaction or dissatisfaction with sex life and its quality, previously versus present.
2. Is there a failure of autonomic sexual response, or is failure due to physical discomfort, postcoital pain, etc. Is the pain genitally located or elsewhere?
3. Is sexual activity in general viewed as pleasant? Often it is seen instead as a duty, and its avoidance is positive reinforcement for pain behavior.
4. Is the couple in question still basically "in love" and attracted to one another?
5. Are there specific inhibitions against engaging in variations in sexual acts or positions so as to adapt to disability?
6. Has the patient's partner inhibited the patient from fear of "imposing" himself or herself or of hurting the patient?
7. Does the patient fear that sexual activity will precipitate serious injury or relapse (especially in spinal pain)?
8. Is the basic communication style between partners adequate for them to express desires to each other, and share personal issues of emotional or physical vulnerability (i.e., to establish intimacy)?

It is important for sexual counselors to model acceptance of sexuality and help patients freely express attitudes or preferences, letting them know that they can do so with their partners. Inhibition can be greatly diminished if couples are seen in groups, common sexual myths in chronic pain are discussed, and options in sexual positions are demonstrated through drawings or suitable dolls.

The general techniques of sexual therapy often suffice for chronic pain patients:

1. Immediate expectation of sexual activity, penetration, and orgasm should be deferred until each reappears spontaneously. In no way should any single step be regarded as a goal, but rather as a pleasure and closeness in itself.
2. Adequate time and privacy must be arranged for the couple to be together rather than to engage in sexual activity *per se*.
3. Specific suggestions may be given in terms of shared nongenital "pleasuring" such as massage and caressing, with the strongest emphasis on each person learning to tell the other what he or she is enjoying and desires further. Subsequently feelings, preferences, and inhibitions should be discussed further.
4. As activity becomes more centered about erogenous zones, the couple is encouraged to stop and enjoy the most recent next step, freely going back to a less sexually stimulating step if inhibition appears. Though no time-course goal is set, sexual function often reappears quickly.
5. The partners need to understand clearly that they probably will have relapses, during which they need to retrace previous steps on their own.
6. Training in communication skills, active listening, assertiveness, self-expression, etc., facilitates therapy.

These treatments are integrated with family and couples therapy. In difficult cases individual psychotherapy may be needed as well. Return of sexual function not only may herald the replacement of pain with pleasurable preception, but also may promote the patient's self-image as a person able to return to other activities, including work. Neglect of sexual issues, conversely, can undermine the entire program.

INDIVIDUAL PSYCHOTHERAPY

In most cases individual psychotherapy is not undertaken as an exclusive modality in chronic pain treatment, with the rare exception of cases with clear-cut psychogenic problems and mainly conflictual neurotic pathology. Also, individual treatment is usually not included while initial residential treatment is under way, because the dependency of a one-to-one relationship could result in resistance to the learning of coping skills. Thus individual work most often occurs as part of an after-care maintenance program for patients who already have some mastery of coping techniques. Since a member of a pain treatment team is usually adjusting antidepressant or other medications, the psychotherapist need not be a psychiatrist, and there is much to be said for using a nonphysician, which avoids reentering the Pain Game. On the other hand, the primary physician, and especially a generalist, can be the most effective therapist of all, if familiar with the pitfalls of treatment and comfortable with some of the primitive features of chronic pain psychopathology.

Whoever undertakes the individual therapy should be well versed in the recognition and mangement of psychosis as well as the rages of very infantile, primitive character reactions. This includes skill in controlling regression and maintaining the expression of negative feelings at an intellectualized verbal level without much uncovering, insight-oriented work. Decompensation in a chronic pain patient usually presents as an alarming combination of short-lived physical relapse and emotional storm. Metaphorically a brief storm at sea is well handled by an experienced sailor, but would result in tragedy for the inexperienced. Caution is suggested by Blumer's (1975) statement that ". . . chronic pain is needed by some patients, in whom it may be a substitute for a major mental disorder" (p. 904).

Probably the most important overriding rule is to choose individual psychotherapy not according to the symptoms or pain syndrome, but rather to the general nature of the patient's psychopathology. Nemiah (1978) points out that ". . . for the patient whose psychosomatic disorder is associated with neurotic mechanisms that are accessible to analytically oriented therapy, such psychotherapeutic techniques may produce a significant and permanent change for the better. On the other hand, if the somatic illness . . . stems from serious characterological deficits . . . supportive and other psychotherapeutic measures are recommended" (p. 36).

Overall there is very little risk and much to be gained from a guiding supportive therapy undertaken, for example, through regularly scheduled visits to the primary physician, with deemphasis of specific physical symptoms and positive reinforcement of general activity, as discussed by Blumer (1975). He further adds, "Such an approach practiced by the non-psychiatric physician tends to carry more influence . . ." (p. 902).

On the other hand, any long-term or intensive psychotherapy of chronic pain patients represents a major commitment for the therapist, who is likely to require initial supervision, even if experienced in conducting therapy with nonpain patients. The therapist's reactions to the patients may be uncomfortable: therapists are referred to Groves' (1978) soul-searching guide for treating "those whom most physicians dread . . . clingers . . . demanders . . . help-rejecters and self-destructive deniers" (p. 883), and the therapist's reactions of aversion, counterattack, depression, and malice.

REFERENCES

Berne, E. 1964. *Games People Play*. New York: Grove Press.
Blumer, D. 1975. Psychiatric considerations in pain. In *The Spine*, vol. II, R.H. Rothman (Ed.). Philadelphia: W.B. Saunders.
Groves, J.E. 1978. Taking care of the hateful patient. *N. Engl. J. Med.* 298:883–887.
Mahler, M.S. 1979. *The Selected Papers of Margaret S. Mahler*, vol. II. New York: Aronson Press.
Nemiah, J.C. 1978. Alexithymia and psychosomatic illness. *J. Clin. Exp. Psychiatr.* pp. 25–37.
Slavson, S.R. 1979. *Dynamics of Group Psychotherapy*. New York: Aronson Press.
Yalom, I.D. 1975. *The Theory and Practice of Group Psychotherapy*. 2d ed. New York: Basic Books.

BIBLIOGRAPHY

Bion, W.R. 1961. *Experiences in Groups*. New York: Ballantine Books.
Cumming, J., and Cumming, E. 1970. *Ego and Milieu*. New York: Atherton Press.

14

Behavior Modification

STANLEY L. CHAPMAN

Behavior modification programs are based on a systematic rewarding of health behaviors and ignoring of pain behaviors. Both overt and cognitive or "covert" behaviors are treated in pain control facilities. Success depends on careful patient selection, consistency in staff reactions, and successful planning for maintenance and follow-up. Results from the Emory Pain Control Center indicate successful maintenance of behavioral changes regardless of disability status with a straightforward outpatient approach. The need for a greater focus on prevention and earlier referral to pain rehabilitation programs is discussed.

Up until the early 1960s, treatment of chronic pain was built mainly on the disease model. According to this model, chronic pain was seen as a symptom of an underlying disease and medical intervention was based mainly on careful assessment of the organic causes of the pain and their removal. If surgery did not seem appropriate or proved unsuccessful, reduction of pain was sought with drugs and with conservative procedures, such as bed rest, medication, and traction. If these failed patients generally were told that they would have to "live with it." In the absence of positive physical findings, a patient often was dismissed from treatment or was perhaps referred to a psychiatrist for intensive therapy.

The disease model often failed with chronic pain because it could not account for the influences of learning on pain behavior. By making patients passively dependent on the medical profession, the disease model unwittingly strengthened their feelings of helplessness and thereby increased pain behavior. Suggestions that patients needed to learn to live with the pain or should seek psychiatric help often reduced self-esteem and produced reactions of despair and anger.

The learning model, on the other hand, held that chronic pain behavior often could be modified by restructuring a patient's environment to support positive changes, and by teaching the patients methods by which they could increase their functions. Thus comprehensive pain centers proliferated with an emphasis not on the medical cure of pain, but rather on directly changing patient behaviors: what patients do, what they take, and what they say. (See Chapter 2 for discussion of the general goals of pain control centers.)

Behavior modification programs for chronic pain begin with a careful assessment of the physical, behavioral, social, emotional, and vocational contributants to pain behavior. Such an assessment should determine if the patient shows pain behavior in excess of demonstrated pathology and whether this behavior is "operant," or controlled by its consequences. Programs that emphasize structuring the patient in the environment to reduce drug usage, increase activity levels, and decrease pain complaints are designed for these "doloric" (see Chapter 9) patients and may be inappropriate for many chronic pain patients. "Stoic" patients, for example, are much more likely to benefit from counseling in choosing and pacing activities more carefully, accepting limitations, directly expressing needs, accepting others' support when necessary, and perhaps learning to manage stress more effectively.

BEHAVIOR MODIFICATION FOR OPERANT PAIN

Because most pain control centers deal extensively with doloric patients showing operant pain behaviors, a typical behavior modification program for such patients will be described.

Programs generally begin with careful baseline measures of significant behaviors. Patients or staff members monitor such variables as the number and amount of medications taken; the daily amount of time patients stay up on their feet; important physical measures such as strength, range of motion, and sitting tolerance; the number, type, and intensity of pain complaints produced by the patients; and the number and type of rewards given by family members or others for pain behaviors and health behaviors. Once these behaviors are counted, the patient, his or her family, and the staff typically make an explicit contract that details the responsibilities of each in treatment and rewards to be given contingent upon successful behavior change. One provision of the contract, for example, might be for the patient to increase a physical therapy exercise by one repetition every day and to increase walking time by 30 minutes every day. A family member might agree to give positive attention to the patient who makes positive statements about such activities and to ignore complaints of pain.

The patient's progress is carefully monitored and measured throughout treatment and standards for increasing function, decreasing reliance on medications, and decreasing pain complaints are gradually raised as the patient shows improvement. Small measurable and achievable goals are set so as to build in success and confidence and allow for frequent reinforcement of the patient. Staff members must be consistent in ignoring complaints and encouraging improvements in function. Some programs avoid use of any pain-relieving treatments during this process. If any drugs, nerve blocks, transcutaneous nerve stimulation, or other treatments are given, they should be administered on a time-contingent basis or given in response to positive behavioral changes rather than in response to an escalation of pain behaviors.

It generally is quite easy to withdraw patients from drugs, decrease verbal complaints, and increase physical activity levels in a structured treatment setting. The principal difficulty in behavior modification lies in maintaining these changes long after the immediate treatment period is over. For this goal to be reached successfully, the patient's environment needs to be structured so that it will continue to support health behaviors and the patient must become convinced that there are alternatives superior to continued reliance on pain behavior. Progress toward greater function may evaporate quickly if treatment ends abruptly with no follow-up; if the patient's family begins to attend only to pain complaints, or encourages taking drugs or seeking further medical assessment of treatments; if there is no vocational follow-up to retrain the patient for work; or if the patient is awarded disability money contingent on continued pain behavior or helplessness.

Successful maintenance probably depends largely on whether the patient has developed enough skills in coping with pain and with life, to be able to gain meaningful rewards through alternative health behaviors. It is for this reason that psychological therapies, such as stress management and training in communication skills and assertiveness, take on such importance. Patients who can express their needs directly and effectively will not need to rely on pain complaints to get their needs met, just as those individuals able to reduce pain with relaxation or self-hypnosis will not likely become addicted to habit-forming medications. A person who learns to cope with stress more adequately is then less likely to become trapped in the vicious cycle of pain and anxiety described in Chapter 15; that person also will not need to rely on pain behavior to avoid stresses.

Studies from pain centers using behavior modification have demonstrated that reduced drug usage, improved ability to perform physical activities, increased daily time spent on one's feet, and decreased visits to physicians and hospitals can be maintained without increasing subjective pain intensities for several years after treatment (Fordyce et al., 1973; Gottlieb et al., 1977; Newman et al., 1978; Swanson et al., 1979). Furthermore, the cost of these programs is more than recovered by the subsequent savings in the cost of drugs, surgeries, and hospital visits (Lack, 1979; Newman et al., 1978). Helping patients return to work generally has been a more difficult goal to achieve. Though these results seem promising, controlled research still needs to be done to determine exactly how much treatment of what type is likely to produce what results with which type of patient.

These results should not lead us to believe that behavior modification is a panacea for chronic pain. It must be remembered that many people report chronic pain that is not controlled by its consequences. Many are not underactive, do not focus on somatic complaints, and do not use habit-forming medications. In addition many patients with chronic operant pain will not accept treatment that is based solely on the modification of overt behavior, but are interested only in direct pain relief. Though professionals relying mainly on behavior modification usually explain to patients that the goal is not pain relief, all are familiar with the vignette in which the patient is told, "You are doing so well: you are off medications, you can walk twice as far as before, you are not limping as much, and you have increased your strength and range of motion." The patient all to often replies dolefully, "Yes, but I still hurt."

COGNITIVE THERAPIES

Partly in response to these limitations, behavior modification has been integrated with other modalities of pain treatment and the concept of behavior has been expanded to include thoughts, attitudes, and physiological responses. Cognitive behavior modification follows the same principles as modification programs for overt behaviors. Thus thoughts and attitudes are broken down into small parts and efforts are made to modify each part explicitly. For example, it might be determined that one patient's thoughts and attitudes are represented in the following self-statements:

1. "My back keeps me from doing anything I enjoy."
2. "When I hurt there is nothing I can do about it."
3. "I have nothing to do but wait until the doctors find a cure for my problem."

Efforts are made to convince and demonstrate to patients that these kinds of self-statements are not valid and can be replaced with others such as:

1. "I can find activities meaningful to me if I don't give up."
2. "There are many skills I can learn to cope with pain."
3. "Right now there is no "cure" for my pain problem and what happens depends on me and my own efforts."

These self-statements embody hope and self-reliance, two necessary ingredients of successful management of chronic pain. Hope and self-reliance, however, will not persist unless they are paired with other therapies that teach increased control of pain, and of the problems associated with it. These therapies involve the entire spectrum addressed in this book, including patient education, relaxation and self-hypnosis, physical and occupational therapy, vocational counseling and retraining, and psychotherapy.

With the increased stress on thoughts and attitudes, programs based on "cognitive behavior modification" have been developed to teach individuals to use their cognitive processes so that they can avoid being overwhelmed by stressors such as pain. Meichenbaum and Turk (1976) have described such a program in which trainees are first given instruction in how thoughts or self-statements affect reaction to stresses; then they are asked to identify the sequence of thoughts and physiological events that occur when they become overwhelmed by a stressor. For an individual experiencing an episode of increased pain, steps in the sequence might include feeling muscle tightening; saying to one's self "Here it comes—it looks like it's going to be a terrible day;" experiencing further tightening and a queasy stomach; saying to one's self, "I can't tolerate another minute of this pain," etc.

Meichenbaum and Turk then teach individuals to intervene as early in the sequence as possible and interrupt the chain through active coping skills. Examples of these skills might include taking deep breaths for relaxation, using imagery or self-hypnosis to distract one from the pain, or making positive self-statements during a painful episode, such as "I know I can handle this if I take a few deep breaths and remember what I need to do," or "I can use this discomfort as a reminder to relax deeply instead as a signal to panic." This type of training has been demonstrated to increase tolerance to acute pain in the laboratory, but its effectiveness in clinical treatment of chronic pain awaits controlled research.

GROUP THERAPY

Group therapy can be particularly effective for cognitive behavior modification with chronic pain patients. A group provides an excellent forum for education about what chronic pain is and how it can be controlled. Problems, questions, and feelings regarding treatment can be addressed. Common concerns, such as why no one can find the cause of pain, whether there is a surgical procedure to cure it, and why progress in rehabilitation seems slow or imperceptible, greatly influence participation and response to treatment.

Much of the benefit in group therapy comes from the interaction between group members. Most chronic pain patients find it very reassuring to know that they are not alone in their problems and in their feelings of being demoralized, resentful, guilty, etc. Groups can help patients get in touch with these feelings and work through them so that they do not become disabling. Those patients who are advanced in their understanding of pain and in their ability to control or cope with it can serve as models and teachers for those who are not. Both parties usually benefit as a result. In addition group members can provide reassurance, support, and constructive criticism for each other.

The major tasks of the group leader are to develop an atmosphere of openness and trust among group members, as well as to guide the group to focus eventually upon hope and upon positive methods of coping with pain. Because groups often take on the characteristics of the leader, a positive, assertive, and expressive person is likely to be most effective. The ability to employ strategically a good sense of humor can be an invaluable therapeutic skill.

STAFF REACTIONS TO PATIENTS

Professionals carrying out these treatments often discover that chronic pain patients can be frustrating. They can hold on to their pain tenaciously, be quite manipulative, and fail to respond to the efforts of the most dedicated treatment team. On the one hand, it becomes very tempting to reject and scorn the patient as "a Workers' Compensation case," malingerer, or emotional wreck, which reduces staff anxiety about treatment failure; on the other hand, it becomes equally tempting to fall back into the traditional disease model and suggest that the patient "try" a new assessment or treatment modality so that suffering can be relieved. The former serves only to increase the patient's anger, distrust, and helplessness; the latter often relieves the patient of responsibility and reinforces a passive role. It thus is important for treatment team members to discuss their own feelings and provide each other with support so that they can guard against these reactions and continue pursuing a course of treatment that gives the patient both the opportunity and the responsibility for improvement.

TREATMENT OUTCOME WITH BEHAVIOR MODIFICATION*

A random sample of 100 patients who completed the Emory Pain Rehabilitation Program in 1978 were studied to determine its effectiveness. These patients received the following treatments: (1) withdrawal from habit-forming medications, if necessary; (2) a lecture designed to teach patients about the nature of chronic pain and the rationale for the rehabilitation program; (3) a demonstration of progressive relaxation (see Chapter 15), with tapes and instructions for home practice; (4) a small family group meeting to discuss how to handle pain in the family; (5) six physical therapy sessions to correct postural and gait abnormalities and increase strength and joint range of motion; (6) six individual 15-minute meetings with a psychology technician, who discussed progress and problems with the patients, rewarded them verbally for increases in function, and assigned minimum standards for increasing physical activities; (7) six sympathetic nerve blocks, five of which were given with 0.25 percent Marcaine

*Published in: Pain, 11 (1981) 255:268 S.L. Chapman, S.F. Brena and L.A. Bradford. Treatment outcome in a chronic pain rehabilitation program.

and one with normal saline. The first four nerve blocks were given contingent on a patient's reducing drug intake or remaining drug-free, and on the achievement of satisfactory increases in physical activities requiring the use of muscles to stand and walk. At the end of treatment, the patient was interviewed and advised by the physician, given activity and medication diaries to mail in weekly, and scheduled for a one-month follow-up visit. Further follow-up visits were scheduled as needed. All these treatments were offered according to a structured team approach in which all team members communicated with each other, shared common goals and philosophies, and were consistent in ignoring pain behaviors and in reinforcing health behaviors.

For the sake of clearer treatment results, patients who received other treatments offered at Emory were excluded from this study. These modalities included psychotherapy, biofeedback, self-hypnosis, behavior modification for weight control, occupational therapy, transcutaneous electrical nerve stimulation, and other types of nerve blocks. Treatment results also did not reflect changes in the program since 1978, including a much heavier emphasis on group therapy meetings to discuss and demonstrate methods of gaining control over pain and stress.

Results were assessed through the use of the following self-report forms:

1. Activity record (see Fig. 14-1). Patients recorded the amount of time they spent in the listed activities daily. Pretreatment, posttreatment, and follow-up results were reported as average daily activity time for one week before treatment, for the last week of treatment, and for the last week before follow-up respectively. (For patients in the two-week program, posttreatment activities were averaged over the last three days of treatment rather than over the last week.)
2. Medication record.
3. Pain intensity rating (see Chapter 9, Figure 9-3) to measure subjective pain intensity. Patient responses were converted to a 0-to-100 scale and were assessed before the first and sixth nerve blocks and at follow-up.
4. McGill Pain Questionnaire (Melzack 1975; see Chapter 9) to measure semantic correlates of pain. The number of words chosen and the pain rating index based on the pain intensity represented by each word were determined.

These four questionnaires together with questions regarding employment status, posttreatment surgery for pain, and perceptions of the program were mailed to patients at follow-up intervals ranging from 15 to 30 months posttreatment (mean = 21 months). Forty-eight were returned; of the remaining 52 patients, 38 were reached by telephone and the same information was gathered, with the exception of the McGill Pain Questionnaire results.

All data represented self-reports of patients. To minimize potential distortion of results, patients were informed at follow-up that results would be used only for research purposes. In addition they were gathered by a team

WEEKLY
ACTIVITY RECORD

	MON.	TUES.	WED.	THUR.	FRI.	SAT.	SUN.
RELAXATION EXER.							
PHYSICAL THERAPY EXER.							
GARDENING/YARD WORK							
WASH/WORK ON CAR							
SEXUAL ACTIVITIES							
SPORTS (specify)							
SWEEPING/HOPPING/ VACUUMING							
SCRUBBING BATHROOMS, ETC.							
PREPARING MEALS							
WASHING DISHES							
MAKING BEDS							
HANDLING LAUNDRY/ IRONING							
DUSTING							
SHOPPING							
WALKING INSIDE (other than in above activities)							
WALKING OUTSIDE (other than in above activities)							
OTHER ACTIVITIES ON FEET							
TOTAL OF ABOVE ACTIVITIES							
WORKING (no. for pay)							
NO. HOURS UP ON FEET AT WORK							

FIG. 14-1. Activity record

technician who had not been primarily involved in the patients' treatment and who attempted to maintain a neutral tone of voice.

Treatment Sample

To obtain a sample of 100 patients who completed the program, it was necessary to obtain 119 records, indicating 19 dropouts. The patients were divided into three groups. The pending disability group (N = 40) consisted primarily of referrals from the Workers' Compensation system. The current disability group (N = 23) already had been approved for and were receiving long-term disability payments, most of which came through the Social Security system. The no disability group (N = 37) included 12 patients working for pay, two who were unemployed but not applying for or receiving disability, and 23 who were housewives or retirees. Characteristics of patients in the three groups are summarized in Table 14-1. As indicated in this table, 65 patients underwent a six-week program while 35 stayed locally in motels and received the same 18 hours of treatment in two weeks.

Table 14-1
Sample Characteristics

	Pending Disability (N = 40)	Current Disability (N = 23)	No Disability (N = 37)
Mean age (years)	38	47	49
Sex			
Men	26	12	10
Women	14	11	27
Location of pain			
Low back	28	15	18
Neck/shoulder	6	5	6
Abdomen	2	0	3
Upper extremity	2	0	2
Lower extremity	1	2	2
Midback	1	0	1
Pelvis/perineum	0	1	3
Chest	0	0	1
Face	0	0	1
Mean duration of pain (years)	2.9	10.5	6.9
Number having previous pain-related surgery	24	18	16
Number undergoing six-week treatment program	28	16	21
Number undergoing two-week treatment program	12	7	16

Table 14-2
Pain Intensity Ratings of Patients with Pending Disability, Current Disability, and No Disability at Pretreatment, Posttreatment, and Follow-up

	Pretreatment	Posttreatment	Follow-up
All patients			
Mean	72.45	52.46	54.80
Standard deviation	17.34	25.24	27.82
N	99	99	82
Pending disability			
Mean	73.13	54.46	53.47
Standard deviation	19.66	28.74	29.59
N	39	39	30
Current disability			
Mean	74.52	55.26	65.12
Standard deviation	14.18	23.29	23.12
N	23	23	17
No disability			
Mean	70.46	46.62	50.94
Standard deviation	16.75	22.50	27.85
N	37	37	35

Table 14-3
Activity Levels* of Patients with Pending Disability, Current Disability, and No Disability at Pretreatment, Posttreatment, and Follow-up

	Pretreatment	Posttreatment	Follow-up
All patients			
Mean	224.62	368.40	390.24
Standard deviation	123.54	133.66	225.25
N	98	98	79
Pending disability			
Mean	221.68	350.40	358.80
Standard deviation	110.26	108.06	208.59
N	40	40	30
Current disability			
Mean	232.59	386.59	439.07
Standard deviation	101.13	114.30	288.27
N	22	22	15
No disability			
Mean	223.02	377.28	396.44
Standard deviation	150.22	167.35	207.64
N	36	36	34

*Expressed in number of minutes per day.

Results

Tables 14-2 and 14-3 present data with respect to changes in subjective pain intensity and time spent in physical activities respectively. The overall mean decrease in pain from 72.45 to 52.46 percent "as bad as it could be" measured from pretreatment to posttreatment was statistically significant at the 0.001 level according to the Wilcoxen test (Hays, 1963, pp. 633–637). The mean pain intensity rating showed little change from posttreatment to follow-up. The McGill Pain Questionnaire yielded a comparable result; at pretreatment patients chose a mean of 11.30 words with a pain rating index equaling 30.85. Comparable values at posttreatment were 9.67 words with a pain rating index of 23.69. Follow-up data from the McGill were omitted because the questionnaire was too lengthy for information to be gathered over the telephone.

The increase in mean activity time from pretreatment to posttreatment indicated in Table 14-3 also was statistically significant at the 0.001 level using the Wilcoxen test. As shown in the table, patients increased activities further during the follow-up interval.

The patients reported discontinuation of virtually all opiates and sedatives and antianxiety agents during treatment. As indicated in Tables 14-4 and 14-5, few patients were taking these drugs at follow-up. Decreases from pretreatment to follow-up in the use of peripheral analgesics, tricyclics, phenothiazines, and pentazocine (Talwin) also were reported. These decreases were reflected in fewer patients reporting use of medications as well as in lower mean dosage levels.

Multiple Mann-Whitney tests (Hays, 1963, pp. 633–637) were employed to see if groups of patients differed with respect to changes in pain intensity ratings and activity levels during and after treatment. These tests revealed no differences significant at the 0.05 level dependent on the patient's disability status, surgical history, pain duration, or participation in the six-week versus the two-week program.

Table 14-4
Use of Opiates at Pretreatment and at Follow-up

	Pretreatment*			Follow-up†		
Drug	Number Patients Taking	Mean Daily Intake (mg)	Range (mg)	Number Patients Taking	Mean Daily Intake (mg)	Range (mg)
Propoxyphene (Darvon)	30	282	29–750	8	272	65–400
Codeine	17	130	64–256	5	45	15–60
Meperidine (Demerol)	7	75	21–150	1	25	—
Oxycodone (Percodan)	6	27	7–64	4	8	5–9

*Based on 96 patients.
†Based on 74 patients.

Table 14-5
Use of Sedatives and Antianxiety Agents at Pretreatment and at Follow-up

	Pretreatment*			Follow-up†		
Drug	Number Patients Taking	Mean Daily Intake (mg)	Range (mg)	Number Patients Taking	Mean Daily Intake (mg)	Range (mg)
Diazepam (Valium)	26	16	5–40	7	15	5–20
Flurazepam (Dalmane)	9	26	5–60	2	17	4–30
Butalbital (Fiorinal)	4	219	100–400	1	25	—
Chlorazepate (Tranxene)	2	40	—	0	—	—
Meprobamate	1	1200	—	1	600	—
Phenobarbital	1	60	—	1	130	—
Chlordiazepoxide (Librium)	1	88	—	0	—	—
Hydroxyzine (Vistaril)	0	—	—	1	150	—
Oxazepam (Serax)	0	—	—	1	9	—

*Based on 96 patients.
†Based on 74 patients.

Eight of 19 pending disability patients contacted at follow-up who were not working at pretreatment had returned to paid employment; only one of 18 such patients on current disability had done so. Seven patients contacted at follow-up reported having had surgery related to their chief pain complaint after treatment. Three of these seven reported satisfaction with the results of surgery.

These results have important implications for chronic pain treatment. They are similar to those reported from other pain rehabilitation programs, the majority of which provided inpatient treatment. This total program cost about $1500 (in 1982 dollars), and provided about 18 hours of treatment, far less than is provided in typical inpatient programs such as that described by Morse in Chapter 13. While inpatient programs have the advantage of allowing for both continual accurate observation of patient behavior and a structured community with intensive daily interaction among patients and between patients and staff, outpatient programs have several advantages besides reduced cost. They allow monitoring of progress and treatment of problems as they occur in the patient's home environment, and they avert problems associated with adjusting to the hospital and transferring improvement from the hospital to the home. In addition patients are allowed to continue work or other productive activities while receiving treatment and are not implicitly trained to see themselves as sick or disabled by nature of their being hospitalized.

These results also suggest that simple straightforward approaches can be effective in chronic pain. Few deep-seated emotional issues were explored; patients were given clear instructions on how they and their families could cope with pain problems; crises were handled by honestly telling the patient that setbacks could be expected from time to time but that long-term improvement could be expected only by staying on the program. Abstruse psychiatric models were avoided and all members of the treatment team could understand and follow a direct course of treatment and measure results clearly.

Much of treatment consisted of reversing previous suggestions to patients that they "take it easy." take a variety of drugs, and continue assessment to search for pathology. It may be that much chronic pain behavior arises not only from emotional maladjustment and environmental reinforcement of pain behavior, but also from patients' compliance with previous treatment suggestions or misunderstanding of the nature of their chronic pain problem.

Many pain programs previously did not accept for treatment patients referred on Workers' Compensation or with pending litigation, because it was felt that these represented major secondary gains that would be likely to interfere with treatment outcome. There is increasing recognition that Workers' Compensation patients, like those in this study, can respond to treatment favorably if they can be convinced that health behavior will yield a greater reward for them than will remaining inactive and dependent on external support. Despite comparable physical activity increases, a higher percentage of Workers' Compensation patients returned to work in this study than did patients on Social Security disability. This finding probably is partly attributable to the much greater income available through Social Security than through Georgia's Workers' Compensation system at the time of this study.

It is difficult in evaluating a comprehensive program to isolate which treatment modalities contributed in what ways to the results. In fact many patients in this study indicated that they were most benefited by "the whole program" or the philosophy underlying all treatments that they could actively

Table 14-6
Patient Ratings of Helpfulness of Treatment Modalities

Modality	Number of Patients Treated	Rating: Very Helpful	Somewhat Helpful	Not Helpful	Harmful
Activity increase	215	48%	43%	7%	2%
Drug withdrawal	114	53	33	14	0
Group counseling	234	53	43	4	0
Life Skills Program (OT)	137	38	52	10	0
Sympathetic nerve blocks	222	22	45	31	3
Physical therapy	221	60	35	5	0
Relaxation training	237	60	34	6	0
Biofeedback therapy	30	63	27	10	0
TENS*	16	25	50	25	0

*Transcutaneous electrical nerve stimulation

cope with or control their own suffering. However, posttreatment data gathered after this study from 246 chronic pain patients indicated that physical therapy and relaxation therapies were rated as the most helpful modalities (see Table 14-6). Many patients in this study indicated that they still were practicing physical therapy and relaxation exercises long after the end of treatment. Sympathetic nerve blocks received lower ratings, though over two thirds of the patients still indicated that they were at least moderately helpful. These results corroborate the need in chronic pain rehabilitation for education in techniques of pain management rather than for sole reliance on physical modalities such as nerve blocks and transcutaneous electrical nerve stimulation.

NEED FOR EARLIER REHABILITATION

Most chronic pain programs employing behavior modification exist as a last resort for patients who have failed with drugs and/or surgery. Since each failure conditions additional helplessness and depression and makes rehabilitation more difficult, results might be even better if patients were referred earlier in the treatment sequence and before more risky or invasive procedures were attempted. Many referrals to pain centers might become unnecessary with greater awareness of the role of learning in chronic pain. Necessary changes would include revising our disability laws so that incentives are given for injured workers to continue working, even if only part time and in less strenuous jobs; keeping patients from continuing habit-forming medications and instructing them to return gradually to normal activity levels as soon as possible; providing physical therapy and relaxation therapies early in treatment (even better would be if everyone learned to stay in good condition and practiced elementary stress management skills before experiencing pain); instructing patients' families to help the patients return to health rather than to encourage pain behavior; and giving the patient reassurance when justified that the pain does not indicate a life-threatening disease and the patient's reports of pain are not imaginary.

REFERENCES

Fordyce, W.E., Fowler, R.S., Lehman, J.F., and De Lateur, B.J. 1973. Operant conditioning in the treatment of chronic pain. *Arch. Phys. Med. Rehab.* 54:399–408.

Gottlieb, H., Strite, L.C., Koller, R., et al. 1977. Comprehensive rehabilitation of patients having low back pain. *Arch. Phys. Med. Rehab.* 58:101–108.

Hays, W.L. 1963. *Statistics*. New York: Holt, Rhinehart, & Winston.

Lack, D.Z. 1979. Multidisciplinary treatment of chronic pain in a community hospital: A follow-up report. Presented at First Annual Meeting, American Pain Society, New York, Sept.

Meichenbaum, D., and Turk, D. 1976. The cognitive-behavioral management of anxiety, anger, and pain. In *The Behavioral Management of Anxiety, Depression, and Pain,* P.O. Davidson (Ed.). New York: Brunner-Mazel.

Melzack, R. 1975. The McGill Pain Questionnaire: Major properties and scoring methods. *Pain* 1:277–299.

Newman, R.I., Seres, J.L., Yospe, L.P., and Garlington, B. 1978. Multidisplinary treatment of chronic pain: Long-term follow-up of low back pain patients. *Pain* 4:283–292.

Swanson, D.W., Maruta, T., and Swenson, W.M. 1979. Results of behavior modification in the treatment of chronic pain. *Psychosomat. Med.* 41:55–61.

15

Relaxation, Biofeedback, and Self-Hypnosis

STANLEY L. CHAPMAN

Because stress and tension influence strongly the perception of pain, relaxation techniques are important in pain management. Biofeedback is widely used as an aid to relaxation and has been shown to be particularly useful in the treatment of muscle contraction and migraine headaches. However, numerous questions remain about the mechanisms by which biofeedback works. Hypnosis is a method by which a person can learn selective inattention to pain. Numerous clinical reports have attested to its potential for relieving suffering, but little controlled research has been done on its effectiveness with chronic pain.

THE ROLE OF STRESS

In our topsy-turvy world, the ability to handle stress has become a necessary skill for our collective health as well as for our peace of mind. Holmes and Rahe (1967) at the University of Washington have developed a scale called the Life Stress Inventory, on which stress points are assigned to life events ranging from 11 points for minor violations of the law to 100 points for death of spouse. They found a much higher incidence of illness at the time of these events as compared with quieter times in people's lives. Surprisingly even major life events associated with happiness, such as getting a new job or getting married, contributed significantly to the emergence of sickness. Researchers now have found stress to be an important factor in an almost endless list of health problems. Cardiovascular disorders, which now account for over 50 percent of all deaths in the United States, have been found to be strongly related in many cases to prolonged increased sympathetic activity mediated by stress.

Stress and tension also influence strongly the perception of pain. Experiments conducted with volunteers exposed to controlled amounts of painful stimulation (i.e., shocks of a given intensity) have shown conclusively that participants found to be anxious on psychological questionnaires or made anxious through an experimental procedure will report a higher intensity of pain and a decreased pain tolerance in comparison with their more relaxed counterparts.

High anxiety levels and muscular tightness are frequently encountered in chronic pain as well. Pain itself is stressful and many patients tense their muscles as if to brace themselves against further pain. Often a very destructive closed feedback loop, known as the "vicious cycle of pain and anxiety," is set in motion; in this cycle pain leads to increased anxiety and tension, which then occasions greater pain, causing still more tension and anxiety. If this situation continues for long, the beleaguered patient is likely to feel helpless and resigned and perhaps to initiate a frantic search for tranquilizers or other "pain-killing drugs" that mask the problem temporarily.

Tension and chronic pain can be symptoms of an inability to deal with a crisis of a difficult life situation; however, some patients continually make themselves tense regardless of current circumstances. These patients may see themselves as inadequate to deal with everyday occurrences in life, or they may have deep-seated irrational fears that something might happen with which they would be unable to cope. As discussed in Chapter 6, patients unable to cope with life may find that chronic pain complaints allow a socially acceptable escape from stress or responsibility. In each of these situations, merely applying relaxation techniques without helping the patient work through and change his or her irrational fears or inadequacies may be akin to applying a Band-Aid to a massive hemorrhage.

RELAXATION TECHNIQUES

While they are not cure-alls for chronic pain, techniques of relaxation have an important place to occupy in its management. Relaxation procedures can relieve chronic muscular tension that produces spasms, headaches, and other muscular pains. They allow patients to increase blood supply to painful areas, which helps to remove fatigue metabolites. Painful intestinal disorders, such as ulcers and colitis, often can be relieved as relaxation fosters proper secretion of acids in the digestive system. In calming people mentally, relaxation also can allow them to devote their energy to productive pursuits rather than to keep it bound up in tension and anxiety.

Progressive relaxation, developed initially by Edmund Jacobson in 1908, is probably the most widely used and well-researched method for deep muscle relaxation. This procedure was virtually forgotten for several decades until Joseph Wolpe began to employ a similar technique in 1958. The basis for this procedure is very simple; muscle relaxation and anxiety cannot both exist at the same time, so by training a person to relax muscles one also trains that person to be calm. In fact, Jacobson has demonstrated that his procedure produces relaxation of striate and smooth muscles and a relaxation in the cardiovascular and gastrointestinal systems.

Though progressive relaxation as originally taught by Jacobson required weeks of practice with each individual set of muscles, the procedure often is taught in less than an hour in current practice. The lighting in the room is usually dim and the patient generally is seated in a comfortable chair or lying supine, with eyes closed. In a calm voice, the therapist asks the patient first to tense and hold and then let go of the tension in a whole series of muscles throughout the body. The therapist continually asks the patient to notice the difference between tension and relaxation in each muscle. To enhance relaxation the therapist may suggest feelings associated with calmness, such as warmth, heaviness, and looseness, and may also ask the patient to concentrate on breathing slowly and deeply or to imagine vividly a tranquil situation such as lying on the beach or in a grassy meadow. Usually the patient is given a tape recording of the procedure and asked to practice it approximately twice per day at the outset.

Patients must learn two skills from such a procedure: discrimination and control. They need to be able to identify when any given set of muscles is becoming tense and then to be able to relax those muscles. If muscle tension has become chronic, it is very likely that such patients have little awareness of it, as muscle fibers seem to "adapt" to states of increased tension. By continually focusing on the different sensations involved in tensing a muscle and then letting that tension go, they teach themselves to discriminate by associating feelings such as calmness, looseness, heaviness, and warmth with a relaxed state. Discrimination of low levels of tension is important, as only partial tightening of muscle fiber needs to occur for a person to experience pain or spasms (Brown, 1977). Reduction of tension occurs in several ways: letting go of increased tension in a muscle allows that muscle to assume a more relaxed state; concentration on breathing slower and deeper calms autonomic functions; and clearing the mind of distracting thoughts by focusing instead on internal sensations and on imagery enhances a mental state of calm.

As patients practice relaxation regularly and thus gain discrimination and control, they usually become able to relax effectively in less and less time. (Patients who cannot should be seen individually to ascertain what is interfering with adequate relaxation.) They then can use a brief procedure, often throughout the day, to maintain a constant state of relaxation. Relaxation is much more likely to be effective as a preventative of pain than as a method to relieve acute pain.

Many other effective relaxation procedures besides progressive relaxation have been devised. In autogenic training, devised by Schultz and Luthe (1959), the emphasis is on the trainee's achieving autonomic balance and reduced sympathetic outflow by slowly repeating phrases such as "my arms and legs are heavy," "my arms and legs are warm," and "I am at peace," over and over again. Progressive relaxation, autogenic training, and many other meditation techniques all share in common the teaching of the individual to be an acute and discerning observer of the internal self.

BIOFEEDBACK TRAINING

Biofeedback training is now widely used as an aid to relaxation and as a method to bring into balance a variety of physiological functions. A person receives biofeedback through equipment that senses a biological signal such as electrical activity from muscle fibers, then transduces and amplifies it and displays it in some perceivable form such as a reading on a meter or a tone of a certain pitch or frequency. "Biofeedback" represents nothing more than what the name implies — "feedback" or information about some biological function.

Information can be a very powerful tool in learning. Imagine how difficult it would be to become a good tennis player without ever finding out where the ball goes after you have hit it, even though you may have had numerous lessons in form. The same principle applies to learning to control a biological function; gaining control of muscle tension, for example, may be difficult when one never gains any clear and objective information about how one's attempts to relax are affecting that tension.

Many scientists have been stunned by the degree of control that an individual can acquire *with* such information. For example, with the help of biofeedback, individuals have been able to learn to activate selectively a single motor unit innervated by one motoneuron in the spinal cord and alter reliably autonomic nervous system functions such as heart rate and peripheral blood flow. Such findings have altered conceptions of the mind's relationship to the body; it is now clear that body and mind exist in continuous close interaction and that central processes can affect biological events markedly.

In chronic pain the greatest use of biofeedback training has been to help produce relaxation. Biofeedback is almost always used in conjunction with a procedure such as progressive relaxation and should be used as a part of a comprehensive treatment for chronic pain, not as the sole treatment. Because success in biofeedback requires motivation and the capacity to learn, it may not be an appropriate or successful treatment in pain problems heavily influenced by the presence of secondary gains.

Benefits of Biofeedback

When employed properly biofeedback can have several benefits. It allows the trainee to learn general overall relaxation well. By observing how one's efforts at relaxation are affecting a variety of physiological functions, one can discriminate states of tension and relaxation. However, it must be remembered that "relaxation" is not simple to define physiologically and that measurements provided from biofeedback devices are very specific. Changes may occur only in certain physiological functions and only in response to a particular set of stressors. Thus the therapist needs to look at multiple physiological parameters and assess how they change in numerous situations.

Second, biofeedback helps bring problems into a patient's awareness and helps motivate the patient to deal with these problems. Many individuals may have thought that anxiety or muscle tension had little to do with their problems and may not have worked at coping better with stress had they not received objective information from a biofeedback device that their muscles were abnormally tense.

Third, biofeedback can help guide the therapist in devising treatment strategies. For example, a skillful therapist may find out by using electromyographic (EMG) biofeedback that a secretary with neck pain tenses her neck muscles drastically whenever she bends her head over material to be typed. The therapist then can use biofeedback to find out appropriate desk and chair heights, desk arrangements, and head positions that will allow the secretary to work with less neck tension. Or a therapist dealing with a person with chronic tension headaches might discover an increase in tension whenever that person reads material on which a test will be given or when the patient discusses his or her relationship with a spouse. This information may guide the therapist to center on test anxiety as a problem or to consider marital therapy.

Failure in biofeedback training can be quite revealing as well. A person who cannot learn to control the feedback parameters may need psychotherapy to correct whatever is interfering with learning. Other patients are able to control biofeedback parameters in the treatment setting, but their symptoms do not disappear. They may not be utilizing relaxation procedures effectively at home and may benefit from using the biofeedback equipment at home in as many situations as possible. Continued failure in generalizing learning may indicate a need for the patient to eliminate stress-producing events in the environment and/or learn to modify thoughts and behaviors that are interfering with relaxation.

Some patients seems able to control the physiological parameters believed responsible for pain, yet they continue to complain about pain. This occurrence indicates that the inferred physiological cause is not determining pain behavior and that other factors should be investigated. This discrepancy between physiological parameters and pain behaviors is a defining characteristic of Class I pain patients (see Chapter 10).

Feedback Parameters and Pain Reports

At the present time, too little is known about the complex biological correlates of chronic pain for results gathered from biofeedback instruments to be definitive for diagnostic purposes. Even in the case of chronic muscle contraction headaches, the chronic pain problem for which EMG biofeedback has been most effective, pain reports depend upon many factors besides changes in EMG levels in the muscles of the head and neck. Budzynski et al. (1973) showed that providing real EMG biofeedback was more effective than providing sham EMG feedback in alleviating muscle contraction headaches, but other authors have noted only a modest correlation between EMG activity and headaches.

The lack of a clear relationship between feedback parameters and pain reports suggests the importance of other factors besides those measured by biofeedback instruments. Results generally are better when biofeedback is paired with comprehensive instruction in stress management (Holroyd, et al. 1977; Mitchell & Mitchell, 1971). Moreover, the importance of the quality of the therapeutic relationship and the mobilization of hope and positive expectation cannot be underestimated. Any physician who believes that positive outcome can be expected merely by hooking a patient up to a machine and telling the patient to turn off the tone or move a needle on a meter downward is likely to be disillusioned by treatment results.

Clinical Uses*

Programs using EMG feedback to teach relaxation of facial and neck muscles generally have yielded sustained positive results with chronic muscle contraction headaches. Electromyographic biofeedback also has been employed widely and with considerable success with migraine headaches and with mixed tension and vascular headache syndromes. Successful use of relaxation procedures and EMG biofeedback with migraines is not surprising in light of evidence that migraines are often related to stress and associated with high EMG levels in the head and neck (Bakal & Kaganov, 1977; Cohen, 1978).

Thermal biofeedback, singly and in combination with EMG feedback, has been employed extensively in vascular headaches. Sargent et al. (1973) noticed a spontaneous remission of a migraine accompanied by a 10° F rise in hand temperature. This serependipitous discovery led them to conduct a systematic study in which 110 migraine sufferers were taught autogenic phrases and trained to warm their hands and cool their foreheads, which resulted in a reported 74 percent rate of improvement in the headache (measured by 26 percent or greater decrease in headache frequency). Solbach and Sargent (1977) published a five-year follow-up study with these patients that indicated successful outcome in many. Interestingly, most respondents indicated that the most helpful elements of treatment were the relaxation exercises and staff interest and support while many fewer cited the feedback mechanism as most helpful. Mullinix et al. (1978)

*Excellent reviews of the clinical application of biofeedback to pain are provided in Jessup et al., (1979) and Turner and Chapman (1982).

have shown that both real and sham biofeedback to teach increases in finger temperature are effective in reducing migraine headaches, and with no differences between them. This result suggests the importance of placebo or nonspecific effects.

While thermal biofeedback was originally expected to work by decreasing blood flow through cranial vessels, it is now apparent that such a decrease does not occur. Hand warming is now seen as a correlate of decreased arousal of the sympathetic nervous system and thus of relaxation. Findings that thermal biofeedback may not be as helpful in migraines with no demonstrable relationship to stress and anxiety fit this belief. The utility of this modality also is limited by the difficulty of patients with already warm hands to raise temperature substantially.

Electromyographic and thermal biofeedback are considered preventatives for migraines. Most migraines occur without reliable warning signs and thus the sufferer must attempt to control physiological functions on a 24-hour-per-day basis. Recent reports suggest that migraine sufferers might be able to abort as well as prevent headaches by learning to constrict the cranial arteries known to become dilated during a headache attack. Such constriction actually involves *increased* sympathetic activity and thus is physiologically opposite of hand warming. This procedure involves placing a plethysmograph over the artery and measuring the amplitude of the pulse with each heartbeat. Several authors have found that subjects can learn to constrict these arteries at will and by doing so control headaches more effectively than control groups taught relaxation procedures (Zamani, 1975), or vasoconstriction of the fingers (Friar & Beatty, 1976), or given thermal biofeedback (Feuerstein, et al., 1976). However, with the absence of follow-up data and the general scarcity of research on this mode of biofeedback, the technique must still be regarded as experimental.

Because of the hypothesized close relationship between muscle tension and many chronic pain problems, EMG biofeedback training has been applied to other problems besides headache. Though it has been used widely for tension and spasm reduction in a variety of muscles, few results of this technique have been published. With low back pain, the applicability of biofeedback is not clear, with investigators in conflict about whether chronic low back pain patients show higher or lower tension than normals in the muscles of the back, as recorded from surface placement of electrodes. (Even in individuals with high levels of tension, it is not necessarily true that the tension is *causing* the pain.)

Nouwen and Solinger (1979) found that 20 sessions of EMG biofeedback training were successful in reducing chronic low back pain and EMG levels in contrast to a no-treatment control condition. However, their three-month follow-up results yielded maintenance of pain relief without maintenance of lowered EMG, again suggesting the importance of other factors besides EMG levels. The authors attributed continued reductions in pain at follow-up to a feeling of self-control over the pain achieved by subjects who initially reduced EMG levels successfully.

The utility of electroencephalographic (EEG) biofeedback for chronic pain remains unproven despite considerable initial enthusiasm based on the findings of very predominant alpha-wave activity in yogis with extremely high pain tolerances. While Coger and Werbach (1975) reported some increases in pain tolerance among chronic pain patients given 30 sessions of EEG biofeedback training to increase alpha activity, Melzack and Perry's (1975) results showed that such training produced results no better than those produced with suggestion and relaxation.

In summary, more questions remain than there are answers about biofeedback training for chronic pain. For no disorder can it be said that the physiological parameter being measured has proved to have a clear and direct relationship to the symptom. The mechanism by which biofeedback works when effective also is unclear. Do symptoms improve with biofeedback because the trainee learns a general relaxation skill, or modifies a specific physiological parameter, or because the trainee's hope and positive expectation have been mobilized? Certainly the feeling of accomplishment that chronic pain sufferers experience when they see they can control a physiological parameter that might help alleviate the pain is highly therapeutic in itself.

Fortunately biofeedback research allows the gathering of highly specific data that will help answer the above questions. However, the lack of a clear taxonomy for chronic pain presents a major obstacle to the researcher, who needs to define subject populations with precision and accuracy.

HYPNOSIS

Like biofeedback and relaxation, hypnosis is a method by which individuals can alter their perception of pain by altering their state of mind. A person does not reduce pain just through relaxation, however, but also by selective inattention to nociception.

Exactly what hypnosis is and how and why it works is unclear and is the subject of heated debate. Kroger (1977), whose textbook on hypnosis is one of the most authoritative reviews, wrote, ". . . hypnosis cannot be explained by any single factor . . . because, like any behavioral process it cross-fertilizes with many areas of human thinking. A complete theory of hypnosis is not available to gain wide acceptance" (p. 32). Research to date has elucidated more clearly what hypnosis is *not* than what hypnosis is. Hypnosis clearly does not represent a sleep state or a state of unconsciousness. The ability of individuals to relieve pain with hypnosis is not dependent on their being gullible or submissive (Kroger, 1977), and does not represent mere cooperation with the therapist. Evans and

Orne (1971) found reliable differences in response between hypnotized subjects and those asked to simulate a hypnotic state. Orne's (1976) study contradicts the theory that pain relief with hypnosis is a mere placebo reaction; he found a high association between relief of experimental pain following hypnosis and following administration of placebo medication only in individuals *low* in hypnotizability. Moreover, Hilgard and Hilgard (1975) have indicated that hypnosis is not the same as relaxation, and can be achieved under states of high muscle tension, such as while riding a bicycle. The ability of hypnotized subjects to reduce experimental pain is not reversed by the endorphin antagonist naloxone (Goldstein, 1980), indicating that hypnosis apparently does not provide pain relief through stimulation of endorphin secretion.

Hypnosis clearly does represent a kind of selective attention and inattention. Individuals when in a hypnotic state become so riveted on a particular thought or precept that they become unaware of others that are based on previous learning and may conflict. For example, a person faced with a chocolate cake might be able to experience how wonderful it would feel to weigh less without experiencing how good the cake might taste. Rather than representing a bizarre or mystical state, hypnosis is similar to the experience of being "lost" in a movie, book, or daydream and thus largely unaware of other stimuli in the environment. "Hypnotized" persons often report profound mental relaxation and rich imaginative or fantastic experiences that allow then to transform their perception of reality.

People vary widely in their ability to enter into such a state. Hilgard and Hilgard (1975) have reported that a person's "hypnotizability," or ability to experience perceptual changes with a hypnotic induction, is as stable a trait as is intelligence. Tests on volunteers exposed to painful stimuli of controlled intensities indicate that highly hypnotizable subjects are able to reduce their pain substantially following a hypnotic induction while those with low levels of hypnotizability are capable only of small amounts of pain reduction. In clinical practice, however, patients should not be excluded from treatment on the basis of assumed low hypnotizability, as they often can be taught to develop their hypnotic skills.

Learning Autohypnosis for Chronic Pain Relief

Countless studies have indicated that many individuals can use hypnosis to reduce acute pain substantially regardless of whether the source of pain is presented in a research laboratory or comes from within the individual, as the pain experienced during delivery or following a ski accident. In chronic pain, however, achieving pain relief with hypnosis is more difficult. One must learn "autohypnosis," or the ability to induce a state of hypnosis and provide suggestions for pain relief by one's self and for one's self. In addition one must find ways to relieve pain for indefinite periods of time while still carrying on activities of daily living.

Experts in hypnosis generally agree that many individuals can learn these skills well enough to provide significant relief of discomfort; however, very few patients have eliminated chronic pain with autohypnosis. As in the case of relaxation training, continually practicing a successful procedure at home facilitates self-control. By listening frequently to a personalized tape recording of a successful hypnotic procedure, many patients can learn gradually to produce the same benefits without the tape in a matter of seconds. Many hypnotists (or "operators," as they frequently now are called) also facilitate self-control through the use of posthypnotic suggestions or suggestions presented during hypnosis that the subject can reenter a hypnotic state in the future in response to a self-induced cue.

Techniques of Hypnosis

In using hypnosis clinically, it is advisable to allay patients' fears about it. Many require reassurance because they believe fallaciously that they will be under the operator's control or that they may never come out of the hypnotic state. Modern use of hypnosis is based largely on collaboration between the operator and the subject. Rather than being an authoritarian figure who tells subjects how they should become hypnotized and how they should feel, the operator usually explores with the subjects what sort of images and suggestions might be used to induce a hypnotic state and achieve pain relief. The operator's voice quality, language, and choice of instruction, suggestions, and images are then tailored to fit the subject's unique characteristics and to give the subject confidence that he or she can enter into a hypnotic state.

Countless procedures for inducing a hypnotic state can be employed and the reader is referred to Kroger (1977) for guidelines and examples. The goal of an induction is to bring subjects into a state of focused awareness that will allow them to respond to suggestions of pain relief. The number of possible suggestions for pain relief are limitless; those that fit with the way an individual visualizes or senses discomfort are most likely to be successful. The patient may be able to see the pain as being attributable to some concrete causal factor and to alter that factor. For example, one patient with a chronic throbbing headache imagined that the pain was caused by drummers inside his head in a never-ending parade. With hypnosis he was able to visualize those drummers walking further and further away from him, and his pain reduced correspondingly. The possibilities for transforming pain are endless: a patient with back pain can imagine someone tugging less strongly on ropes inside his or her back; any type of pain can be seen as nervous energy being transmitted to the brain that can be turned down or off by switches that control its flow.

Other patients are able to relieve pain under hypnosis by changing its nature or location; a severe wrenching back pain can be transformed to a mild tingling sensation. Another technique involves having patients dissociate themselves from pain so that it is no longer part of the body. For example, a patient with arm pain might be able to imagine that the arm is severed from the body and is sitting on a nearby table. Another dissociative technique takes advantage of the ability under hypnosis to recapture old memories vividly. A subject can be asked to remember a happy relaxed time when there was no pain or to recapture the pain relief experienced following an effective medical treatment, such as by experiencing sensations of an anesthetic seeping into the painful area.

Research Findings

Many case studies and clinical reports have documented successful remediation of chronic pain with hypnosis, but there is a general paucity of research findings. Sachs, et al. (1977) described a hypnotic self-control program with eight chronic pain patients of mixed etiology, which resulted in significant reductions in pain intensity and use of pain medications as well as improvement on a variety of measures of psychological adjustment. However, no control groups or follow-up data were available. Their program involved a careful progression from relaxation training to focus on feelings, cognitions, and images associated with pain, learning to modify these through hypnosis, and finally learning to use autohypnosis rapidly and across a number of different situations.

Harding (1967) reported treating 90 intractable migraine headache patients with four to seven hypnotic training sessions averaging 30 minutes in length and reported that 30 percent achieved complete relief of their headaches and 32 percent achieved "moderate relief." As in the Sachs et al. study, the lack of control groups and follow-up data preclude an understanding of what the active ingredients of treatment were and how lasting were the benefits.

In summary, hypnosis appears to be a promising avenue of chronic pain management, but the present state of knowledge and understanding presents few answers and infinite questions. No one knows precisely how hypnosis works or with what types of patients and chronic medical problems hypnotic procedures are likely to be most effective. Hypnosis needs to be used with caution in patients with progressive diseases, as covering up acute pains can result in a faulty medical diagnosis.

REFERENCES

Bakal, D.A., and Kaganov, J.A. 1977. Muscle contraction and migraine headache: Physiologic comparison. *Headache* 17:208–214.

Brown, B.B. 1977. *Stress and the Art of Biofeedback.* New York: Harper & Row.

Budzynski, T., Stoyva, J., Adler, C.S., and Mullaney, D.J. 1973. EMG biofeedback and tension headache: A controlled outcome study. *Psychosomat. Med.* 35:484–496.

Coger, R., and Werbach, M. 1975. Attention, anxiety, and the effects of learned enhancement of EEG alpha in chronic pain: A pilot study in biofeedback. In *Pain Research and Treatment,* (Ed.). AB.L. Crue, Jr., New York: Academic Press.

Cohen, M.J. 1978. Psychophysiological studies of headache: Is there similarity between migraine and muscle contraction headaches? *Headache* 18:189–196.

Evans, F.J., and Orne, M.T. 1971. The disappearing hypnotist: The use of simulating subjects to evaluate how subjects perceive experimental procedures. *Int. J. Clin. Exp. Hypnosis* 19:277–296.

Feuerstein, M., Adams, H.E., and Beiman, I. 1976. Cephalic vasomotor and electromyographic feedback in the treatment of combined muscle contraction and migraine headaches in a geriatric case. *Headache* 16:232–237.

Friar, L.R., and Beatty, J. 1976. Migraine: Management by trained control of vasoconstriction. *J. Consult. Clin. Psychol.* 44:46–53.

Goldstein, A. 1980. Endorphins as pain regulators: Reality or fantasy? Presented at the Second Annual Meeting, American Pain Society, New York, Sept. 5.

Harding, C.H. 1967. Hypnosis in the treatment of migraine. In *Hypnosis and Psychosomatic Medicine,* J. Lassner (Ed.). New York: Springer-Verlag, pp. 131–134.

Hilgard, E.R., and Hilgard, J.R. 1975. *Hypnosis in the Relief of Pain.* Los Altos, Calif. Kaufman Press.

Holmes, T.H., and Rahe, R.H. 1967. The social readjustment rating scale. *J. Psychosomat. Res.* 1:121–133.

Holroyd, K.A., Andrasik, F., and Westbrook, T. 1977. *Cognit. Therap. Res.* 1:121–133.

Jacobson, E. 1958. *Progressive Relaxation.* Chicago: University of Chicago Press.

Jessup, B.A., Neufeld, R.W.J., and Merskey, H. 1979. Biofeedback therapy for headache and other pain: an evaluative review. *Pain* 7:225–270.

Kroger, W.S. 1977. *Clinical and Experimental Hypnosis,* 2d ed. Philadelphia: J.P. Lippincott.

Melzack, R., and Perry, C. 1975. Self-regulation of pain: The use of alpha-feedback and hypnotic training for the control of chronic pain. *Exp. Neurol.* 46:453–469.

Mitchell, K.R., and Mitchell, D.M. 1971. Migraine: An exploratory treatment application of programmed behavior therapy techniques. *J. Psychosomat. Res.* 15:137–157.

Mullinix, J.M., Norton, B.J., Hack, S., and Fishman, M.A. 1978. Skin temperature biofeedback and migraine. *Headache* 17:242–244.

Nouwen, A., and Solinger, J.W. 1979. The effectiveness of EMG biofeedback training in low back pain. *Biofeedback Self-Regul.* 4:103–111.

Orne, M.T. 1976. Mechanisms of hypnotic pain control. In *Advances in Pain Research and therapy,* J.J. Bonica and D. Albe-Fessard (Eds.). New York: Raven Press, pp. 717–726.

Sachs, L.B., Feuerstein, M., and Vitale, J.H. 1977. Hypnotic self-regulation of chronic pain. *Am. J. Clin. Hypnosis* 20:106–113.

Sargent, J.D., Green, E.E., and Walters, E.D. 1973. Preliminary report on the use of autogenic feedback training in the treatment of migraine and tension headaches. *Psychosomat. Med.* 35:129–135.

Schultz, J.H., and Luthe, W. 1959. *Autogenic Training.* New York: Grune & Stratton.

Solbach, P., and Sargent, J.D. 1977. A follow-up evaluation of the Menninger pilot migraine study using thermal training. *Headache* 17:198–202.

Turner, J.A., and Chapman, C.R. 1982. Psychological interventions for chronic pain: a critical review. I. Relaxation training and biofeedback. *Pain* 12:1–21.

Wolpe, J. 1958. *Psychotherapy by Reciprocal Inhibition.* Stanford, Calif.: Stanford University Press.

Zamani, R. 1975. Treatment of migraine headache: Biofeedback versus deep-muscle relaxation. Unpublished manuscript, University of Minnesota.

16

Acupuncture: Oriental Teaching and Western Findings

STEVEN F. BRENA

China's acupuncture is a time-honored branch of oriental folk medicine, mainly based on Oriental esoteric doctrines, held in common by the Hindus and the Chinese. Western research has confirmed some of the Oriental teaching regarding acupuncture and yoga exercises for physical and mental health. However, Western science presently regards acupuncture mainly as a technique of hyperstimulation analgesia for pain control. Data in support of this point of view are briefly discussed. The use of acupuncture in various pain states is mentioned, with reference to classic "twisting of the needles" and modern electroacupuncture.

The origin of Chinese acupuncture is lost in antiquity; it probably developed from Oriental folk medicine and has many aspects in common with other Oriental traditions, such as yoga teaching and Persian medicine. Acupuncture, however, is unique to Chinese medicine. It was introduced to the West by Jesuit missionaries returning from Peking in the 17th century. Since that time it has enjoyed various periods of popularity in continental Europe; during the 19th century a number of books on acupuncture were printed in Italy by several academicians such as Professor A. Riberi, head of the department of surgery at the University of Turin (Roccia, 1974). In the 20th century, Soulie-de-Morant published his monumental work *L'Acupuncture Chinoise* (1939), which promoted widespread revival of clinical practice and teaching on acupuncture in several medical schools throughout continental Europe. The trip of President Nixon to China in 1972 suddenly again put acupuncture in the limelight of medical curiosity and landed it on the shores of scientific America.

ACUPUNCTURE: FICTION OR REALITY

The Orientals did not accept the Cartesian dualism between body and mind; over the centuries they were able to develop a system of knowledge that postulates an existential unity of body, mind, and soul. The typical Western "scientific method" of research requires the experimenter to be separated from the object of experimentation, in order to achieve an "objective evidence" of sensory reality; on the contrary, the Orientals believed in a subjective science, which postulates that reality can be known through a personal, intuitive experience.

Of course, the Oriental method provides a different kind of bias than the Western model, and lacks precise instruments to measure the extrasensory fields of subjective perception. To the Cartesian scientist used to precise protocols of experimentation so that experimental results can be reproduced, the Oriental model of knowledge is quite similar to science fiction. Oriental medicine is as much science fiction, however, as is contemporary subatomic physics; actually the concepts of subatomic physics, with its relativistic approach in contrast to the previously held mechanistic laws of physics, shows surprising parallels to the teaching expressed in the philosophies of the Far East. Niels Bohr (cited in Capra, 1975) wrote: ". . . a parallel to the lesson of atomic theory . . . [may be found in those] kinds of epistemological problems with which already thinkers like the Buddha and Lao-Tzu have been confronted when trying to harmonize our position as spectators and actors in the great drama of existence."

THE ORIENTAL MODE OF VIEW

Oriental medicine is rooted in the basic idea that a cosmic energy flows throughout creation, the intelligent source upon which all forms of life depend. This concept of an all-pervading energy could be likened to the Holy Spirit of Christian theology. Esoteric teaching has defined three modes of manifestation of cosmic energy, with different vibratory rates. Listed in order from the most subtle to the most gross, they are a "casual" level, an "astral" level, and a "physical" level. Humans are part of this three-fold cosmic structure; they share these three modes of being, described in Oriental eschatology as three "bodies" interpenetrating each other. Western science has achieved a fairly good knowledge of the biophysiology of the physical body and has gained some insight into functions ascribed to the astral body, which is supposed to express all desires, feelings, and passions; but science has no awareness of the causal body, which may be likened to the Christian concept of the soul.

In ordinary humans self-conciousness is limited to the physical dimension, through sensory perception; in some humans a dim consciousness of the astral body may be present through inner perceptions via the so-called "autonomic" nervous system. Overt consciousness of higher planes of being can be gained only through extrasensory perception. Many mystics have intuitively perceived the reality of a supernatural world, which usually has been described as a vision of beauty, light, and harmony in the numerous reports of "cosmic experiences" from saints and sages of all religions (Yogananda, 1946) and from several nonreligious writers (Boucke, 1968).

Kirlian photography has cast "objective" credibility to the ancient hypothesis of "bodies" of energy surrounding physical bodies: indeed, there is a corona flare pattern around the object that has been "photographed" by the Kirlian process. Kirlian photography could be viewed as "the process of taking a photograph using electricity instead of a camera." The object to be "photographed" is placed in contact with the emulsion of the film, and a high-voltage, high-frequency electric current is passed through, usually for one or two seconds (Johnson, 1975).

Ancient Hindu doctrines claim the existence of seven "centers" for energy storage and distribution, the so-called *chakras* of yogic teaching. The seven chakras are located along a central axis corresponding to the vertebral column of the physical body. On the physical level each chakra controls specific biological functions via the autonomic nervous system; on the astral level each chakra is associated with certain sets of psychic traits and tendencies and nonsensory forms of intuitive perceptions; in the causal realm the chakras are vehicles for increasingly unified experiences of reality.

The chakras distribute the energy they receive from the outside to the three bodies through a network of channels, which are called *nadi* in Sanskrit. Nadi are said to have both an astral and a physical form; however, the physical manisfestation of nadi should not be equated with the physical nerves or with the blood vessels. According to Motoyama and Brown (1978) there is evidence that the Hindu nadi and the Chinese meridian systems are identical and represent a subtle physical system of energy distribution and physiological control, still unknown to Western science, which is located throughout the connective tissue of the body.

Like the Hindus, the Chinese also recognize the existence of a Master Energy that intelligently regulates and controls all living phenomena. In traditional Chinese cosmology, this master factor is designated as *chi,* with both positive and negative charges (yin and yang). The proper balance of yin and yang forces may be viewed as an expression of "cosmic homeostasis," of which the biological homeostasis is just a part of the whole. The Chinese stress the complementarity and relativity of polar opposites: All of nature maintains a balance between positive and negative forces; when this balance is upset, disharmony, disease, and natural disasters may follow.

In the human body, the chi energy is supposed to circulate in 12 hypothetical channels called "meridians." Ten of these meridians correspond to organ systems: lungs, stomach, spleen–pancreas, heart, small intestines, colon, bladder, kidneys, gallbladder, and liver. These meridians regulate not only the function of the specific organ, but of the whole system of which the organ is a part. For instance, the "heart meridian" is said to control the entire process of circulation from the pumping of the heart to the distribution of oxygen to the tissues. Two meridians have no correspondence in Western anatomy: the so-called "triple heater" and its antagonist–complementary counterpart, the "heart constrictor" (Fig. 16-1). Both of these two meridians are thought to control the chi energy level of the whole body. According to Motoyama and Brown (1978), the triple heater would perform the same function as a chakra center, called swadhistana in Sanskrit, which is supposed to control the entire body physiology via the sympathetic–parasympathetic system. All the 12 meridians have terminal points at the tips of the fingers and toes (*seiketsu* in Japanese); for instance, energy flows along the triple heater from the tip of the

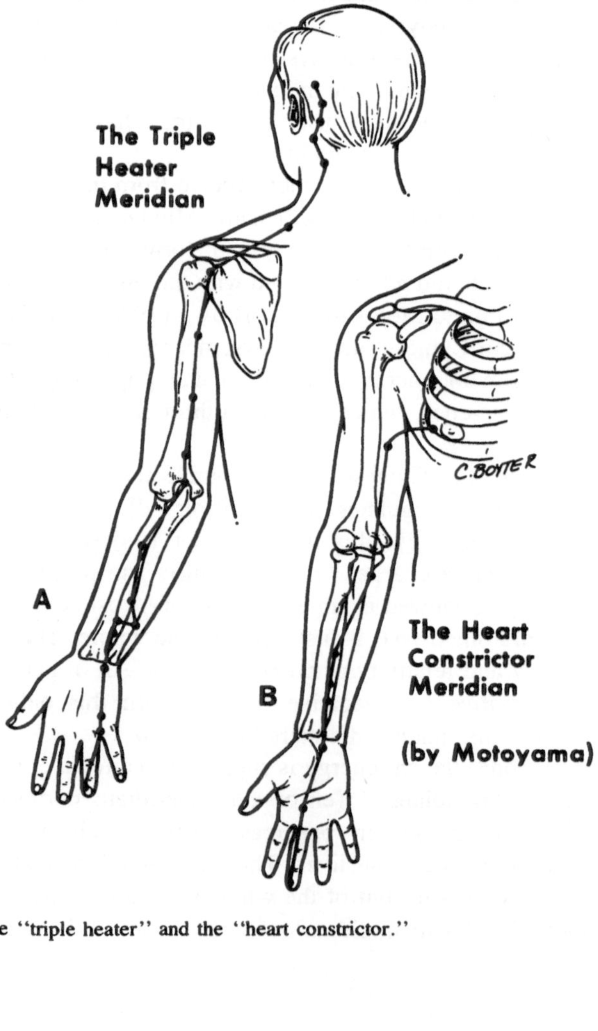

FIG. 16-1. The "triple heater" and the "heart constrictor."

fourth finger to the retroauricular and occipital region of the head and from the lateral chest wall to the tip of the middle finger.

Each meridian has specific points called acupuncture-points, which most accurately reflect its functional conditions. Moreover, there are two sets of "alarm points" located along side the trunk outside the meridian network, which also monitor the condition of the meridians, grossly in the same manner as a voltmeter monitors electric potentials. The frontal set of these alarm points reacts whenever the balance of chi in a given meridian is disturbed, while its counterset along the spine reflects abnormality in the function of the associated anatomical organs. The Chinese themselves do not know the nature of energy circulating through the meridian system, but they have demonstrated over the centuries that this energy can be influenced through the practice of acupuncture and other forms of physical manipulation. Stated briefly, the object of acupuncture is to restore the body's homeostasis, either by stimulating energy flow into a body region in cases of energy deficit, or by dispersing an excess of energy accumulated along specific points of the meridian network.

Chinese traditional acupuncturists use various methods to assess the functional balance of meridians. Many utilize the laying of hands upon the patient's body in order to recognize various pulses throughout the body; some acupuncturists have developed sufficient sensitivity to "feel" the subtle chi flow itself, and thus immediately detect flow abnormalities.

Chinese acupuncture shares with the Western practice of medicine a peculiar duality, which recognizes a "doer"—the practitioner, and a "receiver"—the patient. In the Hindu tradition, this duality is overcome, in the sense that the subject—the patient—takes responsibility through self-training for maintaining and restoring the energy balance along the nadi network. This goal is accomplished through the practice of *asanas* (special body postures and physical exercises) and of *pranayama* (a relaxation–energization technique through special breathing exercises).

Incomprehensible as these ancient theories and practices may appear to the Western physiologist, their basic concepts remain respectable and worthy of serious modern investigation. Two different ancient cultures in different historical times have attested to the same system of energy in the body and in the whole creation: it is difficult and foolish to believe that no truth lies with them.

THE WESTERN FINDINGS

During the second part of the 20th century, Western science "rediscovered" Oriental medicine and mounted an impressive campaign of investigation to test many age-old ideas of the Orientals. Progressive relaxation, which Jacobson proposed in the early 1920s, came to the limelight of research and clinical practice in the 1960s (Chapter 15); actually the Jacobson exercises are nothing but a Western elaboration of an ancient *asana* exercise, the so-called *shavasana*. Meditation, a key step in yoga training, also has been investigated extensively. People who practice transcendental meditation share physiological modifications similar to those observed in highly trained yogis and Zen monks: decreased oxygen consumption and carbon dioxide elimination, reduced rates and volumes of respiration, slowed heart rates, decrease in blood lactates, increase in skin resistance, and a pattern of intensified slow alpha waves on electroencephalographic tracings (Wallace & Benson, 1972). These changes suggest that meditation indeed generates an integrated hypometabolic state of relaxation and altered consciousness, quite different from other relaxed states, such as sleep and hypnosis.

Among Oriental traditions, acupuncture has been the most intensively studied, both by Western investigators and by Oriental scientists using Western technology. The question of the existence of acupuncture points and meridians has been addressed by many investigators in many countries (Nakatani, 1972, quoted by Wei, 1979; Voll, 1975; Brown et al., 1974; Schuldt, 1976). These authors and others demonstrated the existence of spots of decreased skin resistance that fall into the positions of acupuncture points on the meridians described by the Chinese. The differences in electrical skin resistance seemed to be particularly significant in diseased states of the body. This fundamental discovery became the foundation of all modern electronic instruments for acupuncture-point identification and treatment in electroacupuncture.

Other investigators discovered that nerve endings are more numerous at the acupuncture points than in surrounding skin areas and that a majority of acupuncture points overlap motor points in muscles (Liu et al., 1975). These data may have a yet unknown importance for a better understanding and treatment of various back sprain syndromes, where tenderness at motor points is prominent (Gunn et al., 1976).

The terminal points of the meridians at the tip of fingers and toes have received an indirect confirmation through Kirlian photography, which shows a particular shining brilliance at these points. This brilliance, ascribed to chi energy, has been found to be particularly strong in psychic healers (Motoyama and Brown, 1978). In Japan Motoyama (1974) has done extensive study on the seiketsu points; his years of research went into developing a reliable instrument that is capable of translating data from terminal points into information meaningful to the Western diagnostic framework. According to Motoyama this computerized apparatus called AMI (apparatus for measuring the function of meridians and internal organs) can spot imbalances along the meridian–nadi network and thus identify functional abnormalities *before they become organic diseases*. In brief the AMI is an electronic device that records amperage phenomena at the seiketsu points by applying a 3-volt potential sequentially across an indifferent electrode. The raw data are fed into a microcomputer that is programmed to provide refined mathematical calculations of the amperage curves. Preliminary analysis of the AMI data have revealed significant correlates to known disease processes as diagnosed by Western standards (Maxey, 1979). If it is proved valid, the Motoyama apparatus may become a basis for bridging Eastern and Western techniques in the understanding of the subtle human physiology at premorbid stages.

PAIN AND ACUPUNCTURE

The fact that acupuncture may induce changes in painful perceptions is well known; how it is accomplished and the neurophysiological mechanisms involved are still open to debate. Research on acupuncture and pain has focused on several areas: (1) acupuncture in experimental pain; (2) acupuncture anesthesia for surgery; (3) acupuncture analgesia in the management of pathogenic pain; and (4) acupuncture and learned pain.

Concurrent findings by several investigators (Linzer & Van Atta, 1973; Wei, 1975, 1977) suggest that neuronal behaviors in laboratory animals subjected to a nociceptive stimulation are altered by traditional acupuncture; the altered pattern is similar to that observed after injection of morphine. The studies indicated that various nuclear sites of the thalamus and the hypothalamus and the cortical-spinal tract of the cat are involved in the antalgic response. The role of the hypothalamus is particularly provocative as it may indicate an involvement of the autonomic nervous system in acupuncture mechanisms (Looney, 1974). Various neurotransmitters seem to play important roles in acupuncture analgesia. At present serotonin (Yi et al., 1977; Mao et al., 1980) and endorphins (Pomeranz & Chiu, 1976; Pomeranz et al., 1977) seem to be the most likely substances involved. Moreover, appropriate stimulation of certain acupuncture points has been found to activate parasympathetic and sympatho-adrenal reflexes with release of acetylcholine and of catecholamines, again implicating the autonomous system in acupuncture-induced antinociceptive mechanisms (Chen, 1975).

There is no question from eyewitness reports that surgical intervention can be performed with complete acupuncture analgesia (Diamond, 1971). However, it is difficult to separate the role of acupuncture per se and the concomitant roles of other variables such as cultural factors, presurgical conditioning, and misdirection of attention by distraction, all of which may alter pain perceptions during the relatively short span of time the patient is under surgery. The famous demonstration by Niboyet and his group (1973) of a surgical intervention upon an apparently painless horse under acupuncture anesthesia only, and the reports by many other investigators, which show a 95 percent success rate of acupuncture anesthesia in veterinary surgery (Wei, 1979), tend to demonstrate that human psychological factors may not play dominant roles in acupuncture anesthesia.

The rationale for the use of acupuncture in pathogenic pain should be to correct the underlying nociceptive stimulation from the pathological focus, by restoring energy homeostasis. Wei (1979) and others have postulated that acupuncture intensifies the "alarm reaction" of the body by mobilizing hormonal and sympatho-adrenal responses to counteract the biological injury. To support his hypothesis, Wei quotes the elegant work of Chen and the research findings from the group of investigators at the Peking University; he also reports several findings from research on acupuncture effects on blood in humans, which seem to indicate a stimulation of the phagocytic and fibrinolytic blood activities.

The idea of acupuncture acting as an activator of biological antinociceptive defenses has not been cross-validated by Western investigators. However, contradictory speculations on acupuncture findings may reflect a typical Western misinterpretation of the original acupuncture doctrine. Acupuncture, indeed, is supposed to correct imbalances of the subtle chi energy at premorbid stages, before the organic lesion sets in. But in the West acupuncture for control of pathogenic pain is used after an organic pathology has been identified as a nociceptive source. This point may be confirmed by an interesting observation from the work of Ionescu-Tirgoviste and Mincu (1974): they found that acupuncture at the intersection point of the spleen–pancreas and liver and kidney meridians decreases blood sugar levels in noninsulin-dependent diabetic patients, but it actually increases the blood levels of glucose in insulin-dependent diabetes. The authors concluded that acupuncture at the above (yin) point stimulates secretion of endogenous insulin in patients with a still functioning pancreas, but cannot do so in other patients depleted of pancreatic reserve.

Fox and Melzack (1976) compared the relative effectiveness of acupuncture and transcutaneous electrical stimulation (TENS) in effecting-perceptual changes in intensity and duration of pain. The investigators demonstrated that both techniques were equally effective in relieving chronic low back pain in 12 comparable patients. They concluded that a common likely mechanism may underlie both transcutaneous electrical nerve stimulation and acupuncture, and called this mechanism "hyperstimulation analgesia," a manifestation of altered integrative function resulting from the interaction of different sensory inputs to the central nervous system.

Actually the idea that one kind of stimulation may alter the central perception of other sensory inputs is not new either in scientific or in Western folk medicine. In the late 19th and early 20th centuries, an "electric belt" (which was mentioned in a Sears catalog) was popular, and was supposed to "cure" many aches and ailments. Only a few generations ago, physicians used to prescribe "counterirritants" to produce skin stimulation in painful areas of the body. Travell and Rinzler (1952) reported that "dry needling," that is, simply twisting a needle through an area of the body without injection of any substance, may lead to perceptual changes of pain from myofascial and cardiac disorders. Their observations since have been confirmed by numerous other studies using a variety of experimental designs (Erikson., et al., 1979; Brena & Sammons, 1979; Lewit, 1979; Brena et al., 1980).

In the management of pathogenic pain with acupuncture, it is not clear whether the hyperstimulation is more effective at the traditional acupuncture points than at sham points. Earlier studies showed needling at acupuncture sites to be significantly superior (Anderson et al., 1974; Stewart et al., 1977), but a more recent study from Licenia et al. (1979) did show that needling at acupuncture points and at sham points is equally effective. Different observations may be attributable to differences in experimental design, in patient population, and in the acupuncture techniques themselves.

Acupuncture may be useful in pathogenic pain, even if its mechanisms are far from being understood clearly; its use in learned pain is more debatable. By definition (Chapters 1 and 2) learned pain is an illness behavior out of proportion to biomedical findings, in which the role of social influences is dominant. In such situations acupuncture and any other technique of hyperstimulation analgesia (TENS, nerve blocks, etc.) may be expected to produce some changes in painful perceptions, but may not be expected significantly to reverse illness behaviors into health behaviors, unless the techniques are structured in multimodal programs of rehabilitation through behavior modification (Brena, 1972; Brena et al., 1980).

Acupuncture hyperstimulation may be achieved through various means, still wide open to discussion and investigation: (1) The traditional method involves injection and twisting of the needle deep enough to produce a subjective feeling of numbness, heaviness, and swelling in deep tissues beneath the skin acupuncture point (the so-called *Teh Chi* sensation). (2) In high-intensity acupuncture, the needles are stimulated through an electric stimulator that provides a stimulation frequency ranging from 8 to 15 pulses per second. The electric voltage to the needles is adjusted to deliver a current intensity strong enough to trigger an uncomfortable sensation and visible muscle twitches. (3) In low-frequency electroacupuncture, the needles are stimulated by the same stimulator, with lower intensity current so to avoid patient discomfort and muscle twitches. According to present evidence, high-intensity electroacupuncture seems to provide the best results in treatment of chronic pain (Mao et al., 1980).

From a review of the classical writings on Chinese medicine, a general pattern can be found. Acupuncture points on the upper extremities are usually chosen for pain locations in the head and upper parts of the body (grossly within the distribution of the upper dorsal sympathetic outflow by Western anatomy);

acupuncture points in the lower extremities are chosen for pain locations in the lower parts of the body (grossly within the distribution of the lower dorsal and lumbar sympathetic outflow).

Does any relationship exist between the Oriental and Western anatomical sets? Modern Oriental acupuncturists are in agreement with their Western colleagues in the knowledge that both acupuncture points and sympathetic pathways have poor segmental boundaries; but all will admit that stimulation of acupuncture points and block of sympathetic ganglia at the pain location are more effective than intervention at an extrasegmental region. However, remarkably, both East and West acknowledge that estrasegmental intervention may effect the changes in certain painful perceptions. For example, facial pain can be affected both by acupuncture at a point of the elbow, which is innervated by the ulnar nerve, from lower cervical spine segments, and by the block of the stellate ganglion, whose preganglionic fibers originate in the upper dorsal segments of the spinal cord.

In the final analysis, acupuncture, a branch of Chinese medicine dealing with the balanced health state of the individual, has been reduced through Western research mostly to a simple technique for stimulation analgesia. Such transformation has been fortunate, as it has provided a few new insights in the complexity of the phenomenon of pain; however, it has distorted the original intended value of this ancient art of medicine. Traditional acupuncture is not an analgesic technique, but rather a subtle antalgic preventive methodology, useful for spotting physiological imbalances before they breed organic diseases. If the fascinating work of Motoyama and his Japanese group proves successful, Western medicine may be able to move away from just the treatment of organic diseases toward the diagnosis and the correction of functional abnormalities that can lead to the disruption of healthy states.

REFERENCES

Anderson, D.C., Jamieson, J.L., and Mann, S.C. 1974. Analgesic effects of acupuncture on the pain of ice water: A double blind study. *Canad. J. Psychol.* 28:239–244.

Boucke, R.M. 1968. *Cosmic Consciousness*. New York: Dutton.

Brena, S.F. 1972. *Pain and Religion*. Springfield, Ill.: Charles C. Thomas.

Brena, S.F., and Sammons, E.E. 1979. Phantom urinary bladder: A case report. *Pain* 7:197–201.

Brena, S.F., Wolf, S.L., Chapman, S.L., and Hammonds, W.D. 1980. Chronic back pain: Electromyographic, motion and behavioral assessment following sympathetic nerve blocks and placebos. *Pain* 8:1–10.

Brown, M.L., Ulett, G.A., and Stern, J.A. 1974. Acupuncture loci: Technique for location. *Am. J. Chinese Med.* 2:67–74.

Capra, F. 1975. *The Tao of Physics*. New York: Random House.

Chang, H.T. 1974. Integrative action of thalamus in the process of acupuncture analgesia. *Am. J. Chinese Med.* 2:1–40.

Chapman, S.L., Brena, S.F. and Bradford, A.L. 1979. Treatment outcome in a chronic pain rehabilitation program. *Pain* 11:255–268.

Chen, G., 1975. Neurohumors in acupuncture. *Am. J. Chinese Med.* 3:27–34.

Dean, D. 1979. Kirlian photography and spiritual healing. *J. Religion Parapsychol. 20:48*–52.

Diamond, G.E. 1971. Acupuncture anesthesia: Western medicine and Chinese traditional medicine. *JAMA* 218:1558–1563.

Eriksson, M.B.E., Sjolund, B.H., and Nielzen, S. 1979. Long-term results of peripheral conditioning stimulation as an analgesic measure in chronic pain. *Pain* 6:335–347.

Fox, E.J., and Melzack, R. 1976. Transcutaneous electrical stimulation and acupuncture: Comparison of treatment for low back pain. *Pain* 2:141–148.

Gunn, C.C., Chir, B., and Milbrandt, W.E. 1976. Tenderness at motor points: A diagnostic and prognostic aid for low back injury. *J. Bone J. Surg.* 58:815–825.

Ionescu-Tirgoviste, C., and Mincu, I. 1974. Testing and pancreatic reserve by acupuncture. *Am. J. Acupuncture* 2:95–101.

Johnson, K. 1975. *The Living Aura.* New York: Hawthorne Books.

Lewit, K. 1979. The needle effect in the relief of myofascial pain. *Pain* 6:1–83.

Licenia, L.C., Schmitz, T.H., Havdala, H., et al. 1979. Acupuncture: An evaluation in the painful crisis of sickle cell anaemia. *Pain* 7:181–185.

Linzer, M., and Van Atta, L. 1973. Electrophysiological assessment of acupuncture's effect on single thalamic neurons in the cat: Neuronal cooling for pain at a thalamic level. *Am. J. Chinese Med.* 1:305–316.

Liu, Y.K., Varela, M., and Oswald, R. 1975. The correspondence between some motor points and acupuncture loci. *Am. J. Chinese Med.* 3:347–358.

Looney, G.L. 1974. Autonomic theory of acupuncture. *Am. J. Chinese Med.* 2:332–333.

Mao, W., Ghia, J.N., Scott, D.S., et al. 1980. High versus low intensity acupuncture analgesia for treatment of chronic pain: Effects on platelet serotonin. *Pain* 8:331–342.

Maxey, S.E. 1979. The Motoyama AMI-ADP. *J. Religion Parapsychol.* 20:55–59.

Morant, S.G. 1939. *L'Acupuncture Chinoise.* Paris: Maloine.

Motoyama, H. 1974. *How To Measure and Diagnose the Function of Meridians and the Corresponding Internal Organs.* Tokyo: Institute of Religion and Parapsychology.

Motoyama, H., and Brown, R. 1978. *Science and the Evolution of Consciousness.* Brookline, Mass.: Autumn Press.

Niboyet, J.E.H. 1973. *L'Anesthesie por l'Acupuncture.* Maisonneuve, France.

Pomeranz, B., Cheng, R., and Law, P. 1977. Acupuncture reduces electrophysiological and behavioral responses to noxious stimuli: Pituitary is implicated. *Exp. Neurol.* 54:172–178.

Pomeranz, B., and Chiu, D. 1976. Naloxone blockade of acupuncture analgesia: Endorphin implicated. *Life Sci.* 19:1757–1762.

Roccia, L. 1974. Chinese acupuncture in Italy. *Am. J. Chinese Med.* 2:49–52.

Schuldt, H. 1976. Condensations of field force in biological systems: An interpretation of the acupuncture lines. *Am. J. Acupuncture* 4:344–348.

Stewart, D., Thomson, J., and Oswald, D. 1977. Acupuncture analgesia: An experimental investigation. *Br. Med. J.* 1:67–70.

Travell, J., and Rinzler, S.H. 1952. The myofascial genesis of pain. *Postgrad. Med.* 11:425–434.

Voll, R. 1975. Twenty years of electroacupuncture using low frequency current pulses. *Am. J. Acupuncture* 3:291–314.

Wallace, R.K., and Benson, H. 1972. The physiology of meditation: Altered states of awareness. *Sci. Am,* special issue.

Wei, L.Y. 1975. Brain responses and Kirlian photography of the cat under acupuncture. *Am. J. Acupuncture* 3:215–223.

Wei, L.Y. 1977. Nerve transmissions and acupuncture mechanisms. *Am. J. Acupuncture* 5:69–83.

Wei, L.Y. 1979. Scientific advance in acupuncture. *Am. J. Chinese Med.* 7:53–75.

Yi, C.C., Lu, T.H., Wu, S.H., and Tsou, K. 1977. A study on the release of 3H-5-hydroxy-tryptomine from brain during acupuncture and morphine analgesia *Sci. Sinica* 20:116–123.

Yogananda, P. 1946. *Autobiography of a Yogi*. Los Angeles: Self-Realization Fellowship.

17

Transcutaneous Electrical Stimulation: Use and Misuse

STEVEN L. WOLF and VADDADI RAO

This chapter is designed to provide the reader with a broad overview concerning what is known about how TENS interfaces with the nervous system and how this modality should and should not be used. A scientifically sound comprehension of what TENS devices actually provide to alter pain perception is restricted by the limited basic and clinical investigations into this issue. Most of the support for TENS applications is predicated upon clinical impressions from cautious use and evaluation. A host of basic and clinical questions must be addressed before wider utilization of this modality occurs.

During the past decade, considerable evidence has been gathered to suggest that transcutaneous electrical nerve stimulation (TENS) may alleviate chronic pain among patients having peripheral nerve injury (Cauthen & Rennie 1975), post-herpetic neuralgia (Ebersold et al., 1975), pancreatic disease (Roberts, 1978), postoperative distress (Pike, 1978), and labor discomfort (Augustinsson et al., 1977), to name but a few diagnostic entities. While many of these clinical studies appear impressive, their potential value is limited by lack of objective data that have been exposed to controlled and quantitative procedures. As a result the use of this modality is often relegated to a treatment of last choice or to a disassociation from other aspects of clinical management programs. From a scientific perspective, acceptance of this modality has been hampered by unclear delineation of such factors as peripheral afferent nerves activated by TENS; central integration from this peripheral input; and the temporal and spatial responses of brain stem or cerebral structures to TENS. In addition many physicians are uncertain about the potential applications and restrictions in the use of TENS.

WHAT IS TENS?

TENS may be considered a technique whereby output from a constant-voltage or constant-current device is delivered to electrodes placed on the skin surface. This output can activate cutaneous receptors or subcutaneous nerves depending upon the intensity of stimulation, pulse width of stimuli, and interelectrode distances. As noted in a comprehensive report (Food and Drug Administration, 1976), a meaningful and scientifically plausible explanation of how TENS affects pain perception has been hampered by (1) insufficient information concerning current pathways and localized current densities while TENS devices are activated; (2) incomplete data relating current waveforms, stimulation parameters, electrode placements, and pharmacological intake to objective measures of change in pain status; and (3) inconsistency between reported waveforms of current delivered from TENS units and actual measurement of these waveforms.

MODES OF ACTION

Suggested Peripheral Mechanisms

While numerous clinicians and researchers have attemped to address these concerns within the past five years, we are still unclear about which neural substrates are activated by TENS. Most clinicians have assumed that TENS engages large-diameter afferent fiber systems. The input to the spinal cord or lower brain stem (medulla) from these systems presumably activates an interneuronal network that could inhibit ongoing transmission from smaller diameter afferent nerve fibers, known to convey nociceptive information. Alternatives to explain segmental inhibition of pain transmission by TENS would include (1) an antidromic activation of neural elements capable of blocking transmission at the periphery (Campbell & Taub, 1973); (2) suppression of ongoing discharges from peripheral receptors of nociceptive afferents; (3) pre- or postsynaptic inhibition of spinal neurons involved in processing noxious stimuli; or (4) long-lasting hyperpolarization by postexcitatory mechanisms (Zimmermann, 1976).

Interactions Within the Central Nervous System

Melzack (1975) has suggested that TENS, when given repetitively, can alter a patient's perspective of a chronic pain. He believes that multiple physiological and psychosocial factors interact to produce a "central biasing mechanism" through constant activity within neural reverberating circuits. One anatomical substrate for this circuit is the periaqueductal gray region of the mibrain.

Considerable neurophysiological and neuropharmacological research has implicated this area in modulatory phenomena during pain transmission. According to Melzack TENS might disrupt the central biasing mechanism by perhaps directly or indirectly activating pain inhibitory pathways within the periaqueductal gray region and brain-stem nuclei known to transmit to, or receive input from, this region. While this notion must still be verified, it is known that microstimulation of the periaqueductal gray in humans can provide prolonged relief from pain (Hosobuchi et al. 1977).

Along similar lines of reasoning, Mayer and his colleagues (1977) have demonstrated that naloxone hydrochloride, an antagonist to opiate-like drugs, will inhibit the analgesic effects derived from acupuncture. Because naloxone hydrochloride blocks stimulus-produced analgesia or morphine action within the periaqueductal gray region, input from acupuncture stimuli may engage this brain-stem pain-inhibiting area. In addition Fox and Melzack (1976) have suggested, from clinical observations, that acupuncture and TENS may produce similar neural activity patters within the brain stem. By implication, then, TENS may act upon the periaqueductal gray region. Unfortunately to date there is only scanty evidence that TENS effectiveness can be blocked by naloxone in central nervous system loci where neural activity is thought to be temporally linked to TENS-stimulating parameters.

Endogenous Opiates and TENS

Clinical data presented by Sjölund and Eriksson (1979) seem to indicate that cerebrospinal fluid assays for endorphins showed more of these endogenous opioid substances following high-intensity, low-frequency TENS. This finding needs to be verified in other laboratories and should be tempered by the suggestion that patient apprehension or elevated pain threshold may have a bearing upon endogenous opiate levels. Therefore these kinds of data suffer from our inability to control two contaminating variables: (1) psychological factors may influence quantitative essays for endogenous opiates; and (2) as these assays are quantitative in nature, they provide little information concerning the source(s) of endogenous opiate release within the central nervous system.

That TENS may produce augmented peripheral blood flow has been suggested by several investigators (Shealy & Maurer, 1974; Loeser et al., 1975; Stilz et al. 1977). Relaxation of vasomotor tone is presumably more evident when stimulating electrodes are placed over highly vascular areas having a low density of cutaneous or subcutaneous neural elements. To date only one thermographic study (Owens et al., 1979) has confirmed that TENS reduces sympathetic tone; however, whether this is accomplished by direct action of TENS on vasomotor fibers in the periphery or through complex integration of neural input within the central nervous system has yet to be determined.

Obtaining Definitive Information

These observations are of interest, but they provide little definitive evidence for the neural substrate activated from TENS. Recently Howson (1978) suggested that large-diameter afferent fiber systems might be activated during presentation of stimuli from a TENS device. While the evidence was indirect and inconclusive, Howson did suggest that microneurographic analyses might be the most feasible way to gain more concise information on this issue. Microneurography involves the placement of fine-tipped (less than 5 micrometers), insulated microelectrodes into peripheral nerve fascicles of conscious human subjects (Wolf, 1979). Through precise manipulation it is possible to adjust the microelectrode tip so that activity from single peripheral nerve fibers can be recorded in isolation (for a review see Torebjork et al., 1970).

By placing the TENS electrodes over a skin field innervated by a peripheral nerve from which microneurographic recordings could be made proximally (for example, application of TENS to the palm of the hand and recording with microelectrodes from the median nerve at the midarm), one should anticipate seeking a neural response that correlates in time (at a fixed latency) to one or more aspects of the stimulating components of the TENS unit. A conduction velocity determination could then be made and this value correlated to the known physiological properties of afferent fiber systems that conduct at the determined velocity. Such data could provide definitive evidence about the nature and size of peripheral afferent fiber systems responsive to TENS. Until these types of data are obtained, we will continue to be uncertain regarding the neural substrate that transmits input from the periphery or skin to the central nervous system.

THE CLINICAL PERSPECTIVE

TENS Stimulus Parameters and Pain Relief

Generally, during TENS applications, stimulus amplitude and pulse width are adjusted to provide a comfortable paresthesia without concomitant contraction in underlying muscle. When this approach has failed, some clinicians have advocated use of longer pulse widths (Melzack, 1975; Fox & Melzack, 1976) or direct nerve stimulation (Campbell & Long, 1976) to evoke a contraction in the appropriate musculature. The reason for these approaches, other than to provide a more decisive form of counterirritation stimulation, is speculative. Nonetheless it should be noted that Basbaum and Fields (1978) have hypothesized that more intense peripheral stimulation might be appropriate for engaging a negative feedback loop. According to their theory, sensory inputs requiring a higher electrical threshold for activation would evoke responses in the periaqueductal gray and nucleus raphe magnus. These neural aggregates would then produce activation in descending pathway(s) that traverse the dorsilateral funiculus of the spinal cord to inhibit nociceptive inputs at the segmental level. In accordance with this information, Eriksson, and colleagues (1979) have suggested that high-intensity, low-frequency TENS may be more effective than conventional TENS in relieving pain. While this finding may hold clinical significance, the physician should not dismiss the possibility that more conventional forms of TENS may, at times, appear ineffective as a pain-relieving measure because of (1) inadequate stimulating parameters, (2) insufficient duration of stimulation, (3) inappropriate selection of electrode sites or interelectrode separation, and (4) use of the modality as a terminal rather than primary resource.

Considerations in Using TENS

As suggested earlier TENS may be an effective way to assist in pain control for patients with specific diagnoses. When used appropriately the modality may decrease pain and the need for analgesic medications; as a result the functional status of the patient may become improved. Before the clinician considers use of this modality, however, it should be noted that good to excellent alleviation of pain can be provided only through adequate screening procedures. Furthermore mounting clinical evidence appears to suggest that this modality is most effective in helping to alleviate pain that is clearly pathogenic and acute in nature. Patients with pain following surgery or musculoskeletal strain or sprain are excellent responders to TENS.

Patients demonstrating learned pain behaviors after enduring discomfort for some time may respond to TENS when this form of treatment is clearly integrated into a comprehensive pain management program that can include physical therapy, behavioral modification techniques, and pharmacological intervention. When considered as an element within a "treatment package," TENS should not be provided as needed, but, like other aspects of a comprehensive pain management protocol, whould be offered within the context of a contingency schedule. Such a schedule can be in the form of a "contract" between patient and clinician wherein certain functional goals (for example, increased "uptime," decreased analgesic intake, incrementing work routine) must be met for the patient to receive additional TENS.

The Equipment

The TENS units come in various sizes and shapes. Electrodes, wire leads, tape, and gel are also supplied. Although manufacturers offer various models and stimulating parameters, the practicing physician requires only a standard, battery-operated, pocket-sized unit. The limitation on the use of such units rests in the difficulty in adjusting the stimulus parameter knobs.

Electrodes come in a variety of materials and sizes. The standard conductive rubber electrodes are quite adequate for conveying an electrical stimulus. It is preferable to select TENS units that have an insert for the wire connector located at the side of the electrode. For postoperative use gum-karraya sterile electrodes are available. The clinician should be aware of the fact that such sterile electrodes are not necessary in postoperative pain applications since it is possible to select electrode sites away from the operative field. The conductive gel supplied with most TENS units is quite adequate. Electrodes can be taped using various adhesives supplied by manufacturers, but the physician would do well to use regular micropore paper tape since it produces fewer allergic skin reactions. Nonetheless the possibility of adverse skin reactions to tape must be explained to the patient and adequate skin inspection is a constant requirement on the part of the user.

Output Characteristics

The electrical output characteristics of TENS units are highly variable. The physician should consider the use of TENS devices that have the following *minimum* requirements: (1) ability to change the rate (frequency) of stimulation, (2) ability to change the amplitude or stimulus strength, and (3) ability to change the pulse width. The waveform may be triangular, sinusoidal, or square. To date there is no evidence suggesting that one specific waveform is more effective than another. The physician should recall that when electrodes are applied to the skin and the unit is activated, the waveform actually stimulating the nerve has already been modified by skin capacitance and impedance.

Contraindication and Cautions

There are a variety of circumstances for which TENS is inappropriate. The presence of regional ileitis or disturbances in bowel movements serves as a relative contraindication. Application of TENS under such conditions could lead to an exacerbation of the pathology. Gastric disorders, hyperacidity, and peptic ulcers should be considered. Symptoms could become worse after the application of TENS, particularly if TENS is applied to the thoracic, abdominal, or low back regions. Angina, cardiac irregularities, and pacemakers are relative contraindications. The presence of peripheral vascular disease may suggest the inappropriateness of TENS in alleviating extremity pain. Should the distal extremities remain cold or even get cooler as a result of TENS applications, this modality should be discontinued.

The first application of TENS may be by the physician. After electrode sites are selected and the unit is activated, the frequency should be set to midrange. The amplitude (stimulus strength) should then be gradually increased until the patient feels the stimulation. Thereafter the stimulus intensity can be augmented to a level that is tolerable by the patient. The first application should last for only 20 to 30 minutes. At the end of the session patients sometimes feel drowsy. This occurrence usually indicates that there will be a good response to TENS.

It is important to make a brief note on a patient's responsiveness to the modality. There are several ways in which this documentation can be done. While many pain-rating schema exist, an arbitrary index of relief can be undertaken by rating pain according to a relative scale on which over 70 percent relief is successful, 30 to 70 percent relief is moderately successful, and less than 30 percent relief is unsuccessful. An alternative to this method is to present the patient with a 100-millimeter line with two descriptors placed at the extreme ends. These descriptors should read "no pain" at the left-hand end and "pain as bad as it could possibly be" at the right-hand end. Prior to, during, and following treatment, the patient is asked to place a mark along this line. It is advisable to use separate sheets of paper for each marking. The physician then can simply calculate the percentage pain relief based upon the relative location of the mark to 100 percent. Additional paper-and-pencil tests designed to assess patient pain intensity and psychological disposition are presented in Chapter 9.

It is also advisable to keep notes on the patient's impression concerning the duration of pain relief and on the changes in pain medication intake over time. Relief may vary from a few minutes up to a few days for just one 20 to 30 minute TENS session. Most commonly relief lasts for one or two days. At such time the patient should be requested to return for a repeat session. When constant relief is obtained for three sessions, a home TENS unit can be prescribed.

Often paradoxical or contradictory clinical observations can be made following a TENS session. For example, the patient may state that minimal pain relief has been obtained, yet active joint mobility, previously limited by pain, may have increased substantially. It is advisable, therefore, to monitor and record such parameters as active joint range of motion, uptime, and activities of daily living in some quantitative format in order to obtain a more accurate picture of short- and long-term patient responsiveness to TENS treatment.

There are several "warnings" that should be kept in mind when interfacing the patient to a TENS device. Patients with rheumatoid arthritis may claim enormous relief during the first session. But frequently such patients call in 24 hours later rejecting the entire treatment and complaining of more intense pain. Until further data are available, it is well not to use this modality on patients with rheumatoid arthritis. To obtain optimal relief morphine or codeine medication should be reduced. There appears to be a cross-tolerance between electrical stimulation and codeine. Patients on codeine, when treated with TENS, are liable to show symptoms suggesting codeine withdrawal. These symptoms include diarrhea and severe nausea, and may last up to three days after one TENS application.

The technique appears to increase gastro-intestinal mobility. Some elderly patients being treated for low back pain have been delighted at their regularity in bowel movements after TENS and have stopped using laxatives. This side affect, however, is seen only infrequently.

When treating back pain, it is well worth noting that some patients may develop a coincidental kidney infection. Such an infection may even be masked for a while. Regular follow-up by the physician, including urine analysis, should be mandatory.

Abuses and Misuses of TENS

Like other modalities and treatment plans designed to treat the patient with chronic pain, any single approach, offered in isolation and independent of a comprehensive program, can do more harm than good. In this context TENS is no different. Often the modality is applied for prolonged periods or continuously without intermittent assessment of its efficacy. If the patient has been relieved, this improvement may plateau without the physician being aware of this occurrence. Concomitantly the patient may develop an unnecessary dependence upon the device and, as a result, become more reluctant to increase activity levels.

Even worse, however, is the prospect that TENS may not be affording the patient any relief but patient expectation that "at some time" this machine will eliminate the pain permits the patient to deceive the physician about the alleged benefits from TENS. For this reason the modality must be applied for short periods of time and intermittently. It is only by adhering to this philosophy that the physician can truly determine whether TENS has contributed to patient improvement.

Applications

While there are many references available concerning electrode placements and stimulating parameters (Mannheimer, 1978), to date there is no systematic study suggesting the preferential benefits derived from any particular electrode placement array. We believe that for a given set of stimulating parameters, if TENS cannot produce a beneficial effect within 30 minutes following its application, then its effectiveness with longer application is highly unlikely. The physician therefore is encouraged to change electrode placements or stimulating parameters in a systematic manner if mild to moderate relief is not established within 30 minutes. It is only after alternative electrode placements and stimulating adjustments have been undertaken without beneficial results that considerations for this modality should be discarded.

Last, it is our experience that TENS applications to patients with chronic pain appear more beneficial when the modality is used in conjunction with other treatment plans and is implemented as soon as possible following the onset of pain.

REFERENCES

Augustinsson, L.E., Bohlin, P., Bundsen, P., et al., 1977. Pain relief during delivery by transcutaneous electrical stimulation. *Pain* 4:59–65.

Basbaum, A.I., and Fields, H.L. 1978. Endogenous pain control mechanisms: Review and hypothesis. *Ann. Neurol.* 4:451–462.

Campbell, J.N., and Taub, A. 1973. Local analgesia from percutaneous electrical nerve stimulation. *Arch. Neurol.* 28:347–350.

Campbell, J.N., and Long, D.M. 1976. Peripheral nerve stimulation in the treatment of intractable pain. *J. Neurosur.* 45:692–699.

Cauthen, J.C. and Rennie, E. 1975. Transcutaneous and peripheral nerve stimulation for chronic pain states. *Surg. Neurol.* 4:102–104.

Ebersold, M.J., Laws, E.R., Jr., Stonnington, H.H., and Stillwell, G.K. 1975. Transcutaneous electrical stimulation for treatment of chronic pain: A preliminary report. *Surg. Neurol.* 4:96–99.

Eriksson, M.B.E., Sjolund, B.H., and Nielzen, S. 1979. Long-term results of peripheral conditioning stimulation as an analgesic measure in chronic pain. *Pain* 6:335–347.

Food and Drug Administration 1976. *Report on the Findings and Recommendations on Transcutaneous Electrical Nerve Stimulation,* Silver Springs, Md.

Fox, E.J., and Melzack, R. 1976 Transcutaneous electrical nerve stimulation and acupuncture: Comparison of treatment for low back pain. *Pain* 2:141–148.

Hosobuchi, Y., Adams, J.E., and Linchintz, R. 1977. Pain relief by electrical stimulation of the central gray matter in humans and its reversal by naloxone. *Science* 197:183–186.

Howson, D.C. 1978. Peripheral neural excitability: Implications for transcutaneous electrical nerve stimulation. *Phys. Therap.* 58:1467–1473.

Loeser, J.D., Black, R.G., and Christman, A. 1975. Relief of pain by transcutaneous stimulation. *J. Neurosurg.* 42:308–314.

Mannheimer, J.S. 1978. Electrode placements for transcutaneous electrical nerve stimulation. *Phys. Therap.* 58:1455–1462.

Mayer, D.J., Price, D.D., and Rafii, A. 1977. Antagonism of acupuncture analgesia in man by the narcotic antagonist naloxone. *Brain Res.* 121:368–372.

Melzack, R. 1975. Prolonged relief of pain by brief, intensive transcutaneous somatic stimulation. *Pain* 1:357–373.

Owens, S., Atkinson, E.R., and Lees, D.E. 1979. Thermographic evidence of reduced sympathetic tone with transcutaneous nerve stimulation. *Anesthesiology* 50:62–65.

Pike, P.M.H. 1978. Transcutaneous electrical stimulation: its use in the management of postoperative pain. *Anesthesia* 33:165–171.

Roberts, H.J. 1978. Transcutaneous electrical nerve stimulation in the management of pancreatic pain. *Sourh. Med. J.* 71:396–398.

Shealy, C.N., and Maurer, D. 1974. Transcutaneous nerve stimulation for control of pain. *Surg. Neurol.* 2:45–47.

Sjolund, B.H., and Eriksson, M.B.E. 1979. The influence of naloxone or analgesia produced by peripheral conditioning stimulation. *Brain Res.* 173:295–301.

Stilz, R.J., Carron, H., and Sanders, D.B. 1977. Case number 96. Reflex sympathetic dystrophy in a 6-year-old: Successful treatment by transcutaneous nerve stimulation. *Anesthes. Analges.* 56:438–441.

Torebjork, H.E., Hallin, R.G. Hongell, A., and Hagbarth, K.E. 1970. Single unit potentials with complex waveforms seen in microelectrode recordings from the human median nerve. *Brain Res.* 24:443–450.

Wolf, S.L. 1979. Microneurography: A technique producing information about factors affecting cardiovascular control. *Psychophysiology* 16:164–170.

Zimmermann, M. 1976. Neurophysiology of nociception. In *International Review of Physiology*, R. Porter (Ed.), Baltimore: University Park Press, p. 179–221.

18

Nerve Blocks: Chemical and Deep Stimulation Analgesia

STEVEN F. BRENA and WILLIAM D. HAMMONDS

Nerve blocks are a time-honored modality for pain control. Their pharmacological mode of action is briefly reviewed. Use of nerve blocks in pathogenic pain is outlined with reference to various specific techniques of nerve blocking. The special analgesic role of the sympathetic blockade is emphasized and a brief critical discussion of reflex sympathetic dystrophies is attempted. The use of nerve blocks as a modality of behavior medicine in multimodal rehabilitation programs for chronic pain patients is proposed. The possible role of nerve blocks as a technique of deep-stimulation analgesia is discussed with presentation of supportive data.

The first known reference in modern times to the use of nerve blocks for treatment of pain dates back to the beginning of the 20th century when Schlosser (in 1907) started experimenting with alcoholization of nerves for treatment of neuralgia, especially of the trigeminal nerve.

Techniques of nerve blocking developed into accepted medical practice following the work of Kappis (quoted in Bonica, 1953), Mandl (1926), Dogliotti (1933), Leriche (1939), and many other pioneers. Probably the highlight in the history of nerve blocking for pain relief was the publication of Bonica's (1953) *The Management of Pain*. In his book Bonica laid down the basic principles and guidelines for the use of nerve blocks to provide analgesia in various painful syndromes.

PHARMACOLOGIC ACTION

Local anesthetic drugs in sufficient concentration block the conduction of nerve impulses by preventing the generation of action potentials at the membrane of nerve fibers. This blockade is a function of many factors, of which the concentration of the local anesthetic and the size of the nerve fiber are most important. Thin axons need lower concentration than thick axons; hence small C-fibers that carry mostly nociceptive impulses are blocked before proprioceptive and motor fibers. A chemical antinociceptive effect, therefore, can be achieved without loss of proprioception and motor function. The duration of block depends on the firmness of the bond between anesthetic and nerve membrane and on the rate of drug removal; antinociceptive blockade of small fibers lasts longer than motor blocks.

From the early experience with nerve blocking, a peculiarity of such techniques became obvious. While the actual chemical blockade of nerve fibers, as demonstrated by the duration of sensory loss, lasts only a few hours, the subjective relief of pain reported by the patient after a few nerve blocks may last days, and even longer. To explain this peculiarity, Livingston (1944) and others proposed the well-known theory of the "vicious circle of pain." According to this theory, a source of noxious stimulation may trigger a series of segmental and extrasegmental vasomotor and muscular responses, leading to regional "muscle spasms" and ischemia with increased noxious stimulation. By providing release of muscle contraction and increased blood flow to the painful area, nerve blocks may break the "painful" vicious circle and achieve prolonged "relief of pain." Researchers have not been able to validate this theory with clear experimental findings. Moreover modern research on the physiology of nociception has shown that if indeed a vicious circle of pain exsits, it involves much more than limited segmental responses. This point has been emphasized throughout this book (Chapters 1, 3, 4, 6, 8).

Appreciation of the extremely complex nature of pain has led to a marked decline in the popularity of analgesic nerve blocks. Ten years ago nerve blocks were the only nonsurgical medical modality used in nearly all patients treated in pain clinics. Today probably fewer than half the patients with chronic pain receive nerve blocks. This trend in the management of pain is regrettable and possibly reflects failure of the anesthesiologist to appreciate the real value of this time-honored therapeutic modality in keeping with our expanded knowledge of nociceptive physiology and psychology. The performance of isolated nerve blocks for treatment of patients with learned pain without consideration for the psychosocial factors is to be condemned; by the same token rejection of nerve blocks because of unpredictable results following a unidimensional approach must also be avoided. One way to structure the proper use of analgesic nerve blocks is suggested by the Emory algorithm (Chapter 11).

USE OF NERVE BLOCKS IN PATHOGENIC PAIN

Chemical interruption of peripheral nociceptive pathways may be expected to provide significant changes of pain intensity in patients with well-defined pathological disorders that sustain phasic nociceptive stimulation. Various solutions can be used: (1) normal saline to test the patient's placebo responses; (2) high-potency, long-duration anesthetic agents, such as bupivacaine in solutions of 0.5 percent or 0.25 percent; (3) neurolytic solutions for prolonged interruption of nervous pathways in selected cases of terminal malignancy; (4) a glucocorticoid drug, which may be added to the anesthetic agent where inflammation and edema are prominent nociceptive factors.*

Local Blocks

The main indications are trigger point infiltrations in myofascial disorders and analgesic infiltrations in cases of bursitis, tendonitis, and other myofascial and articular disorders. One little used yet highly effective block that has stood the test of time is the block of the suprascapular nerve for management of frozen shoulder (Bonica, 1953). The suprascapular nerve contains sensory, motor, and sympathetic fibers that supply the shoulder joint and some of the surrounding structures. It can be easily blocked along the superior border of the scapula at the suprascapular notch before it gives off its muscular and articular branches. A block of the suprascapular nerve with a low-concentration anesthetic drug (bipuvacaine 0.25 percent) affords adequate relief of shoulder pain, without significantly affecting the motility of the infraspinatus and supraspinatus muscles. Physical therapy with active and passive range of shoulder motion is, therefore, enhanced.

Cranial Nerve Blocks

Blocks of the fifth and ninth cranial nerves used to be effective in cases of tic douloureux. They have lost indication in favor of advanced neurosurgical procedures and drug treatment (Chapter 8). Neurolytic blocks of the peripheral branches of the trigeminal nerve may be useful to control terminal cancer pain of the face.

Epidural Blocks

A report by Goebert et al. (1961) first indicated that patients with sciatica may be helped by epidural injections of procaine and hydrocortisone. The rationale for the technique is the possible resolution of inflammation and edema of entrapped roots in cases of spinal stenosis and/or herniated lumbar disk. The early report of Goebert and his group remained dormant until the early 1970s when Winnie et al. (1972) began to popularize steroid epidural blocks for treatment of sciatica.

Editors' note: For details on techniques of nerve blocking, side effects, and complications, the reader is referred to Moore, D.C., *Regional Block*, 4th ed., Springfield, Ill., Charles C Thomas, 1967.

Thousands of individuals with low back pain have received this treatment. Unfortunately there has been no double-blind study showing that epidural steroids are effective. Because of this lack of controlled studies, steroid epidural blocks are highly controversial and have polarized medical opinion into groups in favor of or against the technique. The controversy is likely to reflect confusion in clinical indications for epidural blocks. Patients with pathogenic radicular pain should be given an early trial with epidural steroids. In experienced hands the technique is relatively safe with low iatrogenic risk. If it is successful, this treatment will return the patient to function in a few days and possibly spare him/her surgical intervention. On the other hand, the same technique is likely to be far less effective in patients with primary low back pain from paravertebral muscle contraction and poorly defined radicular pain, and even less so in other patients with "learned pain" following one or more back surgeries. At present, an epidural steroid block is performed by injecting a suspension of methylprednisolone in dilute local anesthestic solution into the epidural space. There is no widely agreed upon dose, but 120 mg of the steroid in any one course of treatment has been considered a safe limit.

Subarachnoid Blocks

The main indication used to be the injection of alcohol or phenol in cases of malignancy. Almost everyone has abandoned this technique because of its poor reliability in providing prolonged anesthesia and the high risks of complications from denervation.

Sympathetic Blocks

Injection of an anesthetic agent through three needles placed at C7, L1, and L2 vertebral levels completely denervates the sympathetic system temporarily. Sympathetic blocks are useful in changing pain perceptions not only through their peripheral vasomotor effects, but possibly also through the blockade of deep somatic and visceral nociceptive afferents, as they cross the sympathetic ganglia, inbound toward the posterior spinal roots (Chapter 8). Common indications for sympathetic blockade are (1) *upper-thoracic segments*: facial and cervical back pain, ischemic heart pain, pain in the upper extremities; (2) *splanchnic segments* (celiac plexus): visceral abdominal pain—the neurolytic block of the celiac plexus with 30–50 ml of a 50 percent ethanol solution with local anesthetic stands virtually alone as one of the few neurolytic blocks that have been proven reliable in controlling pain from terminal malignancy of the upper abdominal organs; (3) *lumbar segments*: pelvic pain, musculoskeletal low back pain, and pain in the lower extremities.

In the traditional practice of medicine, sympathetic nerve blocks have been widely used in the treatment of reflex sympathetic dystrophies (RSD). First described by Mitchell et al. (1864), RSD remains a poorly defined group of painful syndromes, sharing in common symptoms related to vasomotor, sudomotor, and pilomotor disturbances. In his monumental book, Bonica (1953) subdivided RSD into subgroups, which he called major reflex dystrophies (causalgia, spinal cord lesions, thalamic syndrome, phantom limb pain) and minor reflex dystrophies (posttraumatic RSD, such as Sudeck atrophy and postdisease RSD—postinfarctional, posthemiplegic, etc.). In the early 1940s DeTakats (1943) suggested that RSD progresses through three stages: Stage 1—burning pain and dysesthesia; Stage 2—vasomotor, sudomotor, pilomotor disturbances; Stage 3—actual trophic changes with osteoporosis, muscular wasting, and stiff joints. Drucker et al. (1959) pointed out that Stage 1 is associated with a marked hyperesthetic, vasodilated state, whereas Stage 2 is characterized by a vasoconstricted state that leads to dystrophic lesions of Stage 3.

Over the years much debate has arisen regarding the real pathological nature of RSD and its common pathways. As so often in topics relating to pain, confusion emanates from tunnel vision and unidimensional evaluation and treatments. First, causalgia and other major RSD described by Bonica currently are regarded as denervation syndromes with or without symptoms of sympathetic malfunction (Chapter 8). Second, sympathetic hyperactivity following trauma or disease is not a segmental response as advocated earlier by the reports on RSD; rather it is a generalized autonomic response following physiological changes and emotional arousal. A review of the literature on RSD over the past decade reveals that many known pathological processes have been found to trigger an RSD syndrome: surgical trauma (Kim et al., 1979); pelvic malignancy (Goldberg & Kennedy, 1979); lumbar disk disease (Carlton, et al., 1977); cervical disk disease (Pak et al., 1970), etc. A case of RSD also was reported following myelography (Morettin & Wilson, 1970). According to Williams (1977), the arousal of the autonomic system following emotional stress would lead to increased activity of cholinergic sympathetic fibers on sweat glands, resulting in bradykinin release and Stage 1 vasodilation.

Third, most of the dystrophic lesions ascribed to Stage 3 of RSD are not really peculiar to such syndromes but are common findings associated with inactivity and immobility, much like the so-called fibrositis syndrome (Chapters 1, 7). Disuse lesions are not necessarily only pathogenic, but also may have significant conditioned contributants as mentioned repeatedly in this book. Perhaps the term "algodystrophy"—a dystrophy or malfunction associated with pain—would be a more appropriate definition for many RSD, as some have proposed (Brena, 1961; Morettin & Wilson, 1970).

In summary, according to present knowledge on nociception, RSD appears to be a nonspecific regional manifestation of a generalized emotional arousal mediated primarily by the autonomic nervous system. If so, isolated sympathetic nerve blocks and especially surgical intervention on the sympathetic chain should be avoided. These blocks, however, are highly useful when integrated into rehabilitation programs for prevention or treatment of disuse lesions and emotional reeducation. In this sense RSD may be viewed as a transitional step between pathogenic pain and learned pain, sharing characteristics of both groups (Chapter 3).

USE OF NERVE BLOCKS IN LEARNED PAIN

Interruption of peripheral nervous pathways alone has little value in chronic pain states with tonic nociceptive stimulation from nonprogressive, static pathology, and dominant postsynaptic, central generating mechanisms (Chapters 1, 3). This procedure is even less valuable when chronic pain has evolved into a learned pain syndrome (CIBPS of Crue). Should nerve blocks then be disregarded in learned pain? Eight years of experience at the Emory Pain Control Center and verbal reports from other centers indicate several useful roles of nerve blocks, especially sympathetic nerve blocks, in the management of learned pain (Brena & Unikel, 1976; Hammonds, 1977).

Brena and Sammons (1979) have reported a case of phantom urinary bladder pain of one-year duration that was treated by a series of six lumbar sympathetic blocks, supplemented by progressive relaxation exercises. The patient showed an almost complete eradication of the phantom pain at six months' follow-up. The authors concluded that nerve blocks might have "reprogrammed" central neuronal behaviors by repeated overloading peripheral afferent inputs rather than by blocking nociceptive stimulation from a nonexisting organ.

Brena et al. (1980), in a double-blind, crossover design study, have shown significant mean reductions in subjective pain intensity lasting one month after treatment in 20 patients with low back pain of long duration from osteoarthritis. Each subject received 12 lumbar sympathetic blocks, six with normal saline and six with 0.25 percent bupivacaine. No significant difference was found between the results from analgesic and saline blocks. The patients' Minnesota Multiphasic Personality Inventory profiles were indicative of reduced depression and increased ability to manage their lives posttreatment and at three-month follow-up. No significant changes were recorded with respect to electromyelography of the paravertebral muscles, spine range of mobility, and activities of daily living. Results were discussed in terms of massive placebo effect and analgesia obtained through deep stimulation of various tissue structures.

If, indeed, the nerve blocks produce changes in painful perceptions through peripheral sensory overload, they may be linked to both electrical acupuncture and transcutaneous electrical nerve stimulation (TENS) (Chapters 16, 17) with an added pharmacological action. The analgesic mechanism of hyperstimulation may be viewed as a "jamming" of patterned central neuronal activities "engrammed"—so to speak—in the central nervous system by tonic peripheral nociception. The altered neuronal behavior outlasts the duration of stimulation by delaying, or suppressing, the recall of previous memory-like patterns of neuronal firing.

Placebo interventions may reprogram neuronal activity through activation of various neural transmitters, but their role remains open to discussion and investigations (Chapters 4, 19).

In learned pain the conditioning process deeply affects responses to nerve blocking. Brena et al. (1979) studied responses to sympathetic nerve blocks and placebos in a group of 144 patients with chronic pain of long duration, with no reference to a particular pain location or any specific disease process. Seventy subjects had no paid disability, and 74 subjects were receiving monetary compensation for an accident at work. Among the patients with no disability, 67 percent reported decreased pain intensity following either bupivacine or saline injections, or both. Fifty percent of the Workers' Compensation group reported similar results. Of the group with no paid disability, 35.7 percent of the patients reported placebo effects, but only 17.6 percent with Workers' Compensation benefits reported similar effects.

Several nocebo responses also have been observed following sympathetic nerve blocks in patients with learned pain. A nocebo response is defined as follows: (1) escalation of bizarre and dramatized complaints out of proportion to the mild discomfort reported by the majority of patients receiving the same nerve blocks; and (2) reports of various bodily impairments following a nerve block that do not fit any known chemical, physiological, and anatomical pattern and may last for days and weeks. Nocebo responses seem to be more frequent in patients with pending litigation or actual disability benefits than in patients with no paid disability.

Nocebo is the first person, singular, of the future tense of the Latin word *nocere*, meaning "I shall hurt." In other words the conditioned expectation of a painful experience actually enhances and magnifies the experience itself; hence nocebo responses may be viewed as another expression of "learned helplessness" (Chapters 5, 6).

In conclusion nerve blocks may be viewed as a modality of behavior medicine for pain control and rehabilitation in learned pain states. Several positive and negative effects are likely from this therapeutic modality.

Positive Effects

1. Nerve blocks alter nervous inputs and provide changes in sensation.
2. Through repeated and periodic needling, the deep tissue stimulation may achieve prolonged analgesia by altering central neuronal behaviors.

3. Through changes in peripheral blood flow, sympathetic blocks may decrease tissue edema and reestablish tissue homeostasis.
4. Most chronic sufferers have difficulty accepting the idea that their discomfort is related to multiple physical and emotional malfunctions: (a) by targeting medical intervention at the pain location, the patient is reassured that his/her pain is accepted, even with minimal evidence of a nociceptive focus; (b) nerve blocks allow patients to rationalize improvement as a consequence of a conventional medical intervention.
5. When structured in behavior modification programs, nerve blocking enhances the patient–doctor relationship, strengthening the role of the physician as an educator who reinforces the global goals of rehabilitation.

Negative Effects

1. If not properly presented as a modality of rehabilitation medicine, nerve blocking may reinforce the social status of the sufferer, confirming his/her claim to be sick and disabled and fostering dependency and passivity.
2. Manipulative patients can use nocebo responses following nerve blocks as an excuse for their own failure to comply with the rehabilitation goals.
3. Nerve blocks are invasive techniques with known complications and higher morbidity risks than TENS and acupuncture.

REFERENCES

Bonica, J.J. (Ed.) 1969. *Regional Anesthesia*. Philadelphia: F.A. Davis.

Bonica, J.J. 1953. *The Management of Pain*. Philadelphia: Lea & Febiger.

Brena, S.F. 1961. Les cliniques de la douleur. *Anes. Europ*. 2:230–256.

Brena, S.F., Chapman, S.L., and Bradford, L.A. 1979. Conditioned responses to treatment in chronic pain patients: Effects of compensation for work-related accidents. *Bull. L.A. Neurolog. Soc.* 44:48–52.

Brena, S.F., and Sammons, E.E. 1979. Phantom urinary bladder pain: Case report. *Pain* 7:197–201.

Brena, S.F., and Unikel, I.P. 1976. Nerve blocks and contingency management in chronic pain states. In *Advances in Pain Research and Therapy*, J.J. Bonica and D. Albe-Fessard (Eds.). New York: Raven Press, pp. 707–710.

Brena, S.F., Wolf, S.L., Chapman, S.L., and Hammonds, W.D. 1980. Chronic back pain: Electromyographic, motion and behavioral assessments following sympathetic nerve blocks and placebos. *Pain* 8:1–10.

Carlson, D.H., Simon, H., and Wegner, W. 1977. Bone scanning and diagnosis of reflex sympathetic dystrophy, secondary to herniated lumbar discs. *Neurology* 27:971–973.

DeTakats, G. 1943. Nature of painful vasodilation in causalgic states. *Arch. Neurol. Psychiatr.* 50:318–325.

Dogliotti, A.M. 1933. A new method of block anesthesia: Segmented peridermal anesthesia. *Am. J. Surg.* 20:107–110.

Drucker, W.R., Hulsey, P.A., Holden, W.D., and Bukovnic, J.A. 1959. Pathogenesis of post-traumatic sympathetic dystrophy. *Am. J. Surg.* 97:454–460.

Goebert, W.H., Jallo, S.J., Gardner, W.H., and Wasmugh, C.E. 1961. Painful radiculopathy treated with epidural injections of procaine and hydrocortisone acetate. *Anesthes. Analges.* 40:130–134.

Goldberg, M.I., and Kennedy, S.F. 1979. Reflex sympathetic dystrophy: Recognition and management in gynecologic oncology. *Gynec. Oncol.* 8:288–295.

Hammonds, W.H. 1977. The treatment of chronic pain, a multi-faceted approach—Case history number 94. *Anesthes. Analges.* 56:118–122.

Kim, H.J., Kozin, F., Johnson, R.P., and Hines, R. 1979. Reflex sympathetic dystrophy syndrome of the knee following minescectomy. *Arthrit. Rheumat.* 22:177–181.

Leriche, R. 1939. *Surgery of Pain*. Baltimore: Williams & Wilkins.

Livingston, W.K. 1944. *Pain Mechanisms*. New York: Macmillan.

Mendl, F. 1926. *Die Paravertebral Injection*. Vienna: J. Springer.

Mitchell, S.W., Moorehouse, G.R., and Keen, W.W. 1864. *Gunshot Wounds and Other Injuries of Nerves*. Philadelphia: J.B. Lippincott.

Morettin, L.B., and Wilson, M. 1970. Severe reflex algodystrophy (Sudeck's atrophy) as a complication of myelography: report of two cases. *Am. J. Radiol.* 110:156–158.

Pak, T.J., Martin, G.M., Magness, J.L., and Kavanaugh, G.J. 1970. Reflex sympathetic dystrophy: Review of 140 cases. *Minn. Med.* 53:507–512.

Williams, W.R. 1977. Reflex sympathetic dystrophy. *Rheumatol. Rehab.* 16:119–124.

Winnie, A.P., Hartman, J.T., Meyers, H.L., Jr., et al. 1972. Pain Clinic II: Intradural and extradural corticosteroids for sciatica. *Anes. Anal.* 51:990–1003.

19

The Placebo Response

JAMES ROUTON

Research on placebos has demonstrated conclusively that they frequently can mimic the beneficial and toxic effects of an active drug. Their effectiveness depends on the manner in which they are given and on the characteristics of the subject to whom they are given. They may be effective through activation of the endogenous pain-suppression system. Ethical guidelines for their use are presented.

In many chapters of this book a placebo effect relative to various treatment modalities for chronic pain was mentioned, or at least implied by the lack of a clear understanding of the neurophysiological mechanisms subserving the observed changes in the subjective pain intensity. Indeed it has been shown that 35 percent of patients with chronic pain are placebo reactors (Evans, 1974).

The word *placebo* is the first person, singular, of the future indicative of the Latin verb *placere*, meaning "to please." The first known use of the word dates at least to the 13th century when placebo was the name commonly given during Vespers in the offering for the dead in Latin service. It was not until the 1787 edition of Quincy's *Lexicon* that the word placebo was given a therapeutic connotation when it was defined as "a commonplace medicine." Hooper's *Medical Dictionary* in 1811 defined placebo as "a name given to any medicine adopted more to please than to benefit the patient." Despite the fact that by the beginning of the 20th century the placebo was prescribed freely and the word was in daily use, it was not listed in the index of H.C. Wood's *Famous Therapeutics*, whose 14 editions covered the period from 1875 to 1908. If Wood was unwilling to discuss placebos, it is not surprising to find the subject avoided in most books on medical treatment until the late 1940s and the early 1950s. Pepper (1945) noted: "The giving of a placebo seems to be a function of the physician which, like certain of the functions of the body is not to be mentioned in polite society." A more contemporary definition of placebos is found in *Dorland's Medical Dictionary* where placebo is defined as "an inactive substance or preparation, formally given to please or gratify the patient, now also used in controlled studies to determine the efficacy of a medical substance." The 1977 *Webster's New*

Collegiate Dictionary defines placebo as "a medication prescribed more for the mental relief of the patient than for its actual effect on the disorder."

Semantically the terms "impure placebo," "pure or true placebo," and "placebo effect" need to be differentiated. Impure placebo is a substance with some pharmacological activities not relevant to the problem being treated. A pure or true placebo is without pharmacological activity. The placebo effect is defined as "the effect of any therapeutic procedure which objectively does not have any specific activity for the condition being treated."

Perhaps the early physician did not have a proper understanding of the use of the placebo, or an adequate appreciation for the power of this therapeutic entity. Probably the credit for scientific demonstration of the usefulness of placebos should go to Beecher for his numerous studies on this subject. In his famous book *Measurement of Subjective Responses* (1959), Beecher reported that he was "struck" by the consistently great effectiveness of placebos in relieving even severe postoperative pain. In 162 patients suffering postoperative pain from a variety of surgical procedures, Beecher found that a dose of morphine equal to 15 mg per 75 kg of weight would produce satisfactory pain relief in 75 percent of the patients; of these same patients, 35 percent would also be relieved by placebo. Thus Beecher concluded that the placebo medication was almost 50 percent as effective as the dose of morphine. Similar results are also quoted by Evans (1974). Yonemoto et al. (1975) found an even greater placebo effect: the placebo was 77 percent as effective as 75 mg of Demerol in controlling postoperative pain, with no significant difference in onset, duration, or effectiveness of pain relief.

The same high level of relief may be produced by placebo medication, independently from the subjective state under examination—angina pectoris, seasickness, headache, etc. In some 15 studies from various institutions involving more than 1000 patients, placebo intervention satisfactorily relieved 35 percent of the subjects on the average.

The power of placebo medication has been demonstrated by many others using different drugs. Wolf (1954) reported relief of pain from placebo in a patient with rheumatoid arthritis, which was equal to the effects of aspirin or cortisone. He also found the lowering of blood pressure in a hypertensive patient receiving a placebo to be equal to the effect of reserpine. Hillis (1952) obtained cough reduction in patients treated with placebo that was equal to the effect obtained with 30 mg of codeine. Sturdebant and Isenberg (1977) found that the placebo was just as effective in relieving acute epigastric pain in patients with demonstrated duodenal ulcer as was a large dose of antacid. Hartman and Gobel (1976) compared the effects of placebo on exercise response and nitroglycerin consumption. They were able to demonstrate a 30 percent decrease in nitroglycerin intake in 65 percent of patients receiving placebo medication.

However, they could not demonstrate an increase in exercise following the subjective improvement.

In another study on placebo responses among cardiac patients, Beecher (1961) discussed surgery as a placebo. This study concerned the surgical ligation of internal mammary arteries for the relief of angina pectoris. The surgery was intended to shunt blood to the coronary arteries and relieve myocardial ischemia. Some of the patients had the internal mammary artery ligated and some merely had the sutures left in place but not ligated. The patients were evaluated in the postoperative period by observers who did not know whether ligation had been carried out or whether only a skin incision had been made. It was demonstrated that ligation produced no greater benefit than the sham operations. Greatly increased work tolerance and decreased consumption of nitroglycerin were the common findings of nearly all the observers in patients with and without the actual arterial ligation. The findings of Beecher have been confirmed by other, similar studies (Diamond & Little, 1968).

Beecher (1961) found that the enthusiasm of the surgeon can have a significant effect on the results of a given surgical procedure. He compared the results from actual ligation of the mammary artery and from the sham surgery in cardiac patients. Patients were divided into two groups: one group had surgery performed by surgeons who were enthusiastic about the procedure, while another group had surgery performed by a skeptical surgeon. Because of the previously cited findings about the equal effectiveness of both the actual surgery and the placebo surgery, the only variable in this study was the surgeon's attitude. Out of 233 patients, 43 percent operated by an "enthusiastic" surgeon did report significant decrease of angina episodes and increased work tolerance; these same results were reported by only 10 percent of 59 patients operated on by "skeptic" surgeons. Park and Covi (1965) reported similar observations: a group of patients receiving psychological care were told that they were receiving sugar pills; however, the attending physician expressed a great deal of confidence that such pills would be effective. Of the 14 patients receiving sugar pills, 13 improved in all parameters tested.

Lyerly et al. (1964) performed a study to shed light on the role of instructions and remarks made by a physician in administering an active drug or a placebo. The study involved the use of a stimulant (amphetamine), a sedative (chlorhydrate), and lactose tablets as placebos. The subjects were told either that they were receiving an energizer or a sedative, or else they were given no information. Tests were given for the effects on both motor performance and mood, the latter expressed verbally. The effects of giving the lactose tablets along with instructions that the subject was given an energizer or sedative, mimicked the actual effect of the amphetamine or of the chlorhydrate. False instructions, such as telling the subject that he or she was receiving chlorhydrate when actually it was amphetamine, counteracted some of the pharmacological effects of the administered drug.

Just as placebos mimic active drugs with positive responses, there are also reports of negative or toxic reactions to placebos. Tucker (cited in Wolf and Pinsky, 1954), in a study comparing the toxic effects of streptomycin and placebo, found that of the patients given only placebo, 61 percent showed one or more symptoms of "streptomycin toxicity." The toxic effects included high-tone and low-tone hearing loss, eosinophilia, and impairment of urea clearance. In a study comparing antihypertensive medications and placebos, Shapiro and Grollman (1953) observed that one of the most persisent "hydrolazine headaches" occurred in an individual who was actually getting a placebo. Nonspecific toxic effects from placebo medications such as sleepiness, sleeplessness, nausea, tremors, dizziness, and palpitation were reported by Wolf and Pinsky (1954). Mintz (1977) reported symptoms of physical dependence on placebo medication and withdrawal symptoms when the placebo was discontinued.

Basbaum and Fields (1978) suggested that placebos may induce their pain-relieving effects through activation of the endogenous pain-suppression system. Levine et al. (1978) studied the effect of naloxone on dental postoperative pain to test the hypothesis that the neuropeptides mediate placebo analgesia: Of a group of subjects receiving a placebo, 39 percent were identified as being placebo responders when their pain, after one hour, was decreased. If such decrease of the postoperative dental pain did not occur, patients were identified as nonplacebo responders. When naloxone was given two hours later as a second drug, no change in subjective pain intensity was noted in the group of "nonresponders." However, when naloxone was given as the second drug to the group of "placebo responders," they reported that pain intensity increased significantly, and matched the intensity of pain reported by the group of nonresponders. The authors speculated that such results in the two groups of study subjects may be due to release of neuropeptides within the central nervous system.

Moertel et al. (1976) studied some social–emotional characteristics of placebo responders. They found that patients who respond to placebo include well-educated persons with professional occupations, farmers, women who work outside the home, and people who have suffered a traumatic marital experience. This group has in common a life-style requiring heavy responsibility and demanding independent performance. Pain-induced dependency may be particularly worrisome in these persons, and the desire to reduce such dependency may be an important factor in the susceptibility to placebo interventions. In contrast, Moretel also found that placebo nonresponders include many persons with a life-style that is relatively low in personal responsibility and high in significant dependence upon others. The dependency caused by the painful experience would be less disturbing in this group of persons with a weaker determination to seek relief; consequently they may be less likely to respond to placebos.

The effects of various levels of anxiety on placebo response was studied by Evans (1974). He demonstrated the difference in relief of experimental pain by placebo in groups of patients classified as either anxious or nonanxious by appropriate testing. The pain threshold was significantly increased by placebo equally in the two groups of patients; however, the increase in pain tolerance produced by placebo was four times as great in the anxious group of patients as in the patients with a low level of anxiety. It has also been shown (Evans, 1974) that placebo analgesia is not related to hypnotic suggestibility or to situational episodic anxiety, but rather it is related to chronic trait anxiety.

Chapman and Brena (1982) found fewer placebo responses to saline injections in chronic low back pain patients who were fixed in their focus on pain, showed evidence of learned pain behaviors, and had few responsibilities.

Since it has been conclusively demonstrated that placebos provide 35 to 80 percent as much decrease in subjective pain intensity as morphine and Demerol, should placebo intervention become a routine treatment modality in patients with chronic pain? Benson and McCallie (1979), while discussing placebo therapy for control of pain in patients with angina pectoris, remarked that the remarkable efficacy of placebos should not be disregarded as ridiculous: "After all, unlike most other forms of therapy, the placebo effect has withstood the test of time and continues to be safe and inexpensive." Kadlec (1977) has presented a good review of the ethical and practical problems a physician may encounter when using the placebo. The questions he posed include (1) How should one handle the patient with vague symptoms who pushes for treatment? Should a placebo be used instead of a potentially harmful drug? (2) Should the patient be charged the usual fee for placebo therapy? (3) Is the physician deceiving the patient when using a placebo? The authors encouraged physicians to recognize the usefulness of placebo effects and to keep an open mind concerning their use.

Obviously the ethical dimension of placebo therapy remains controversial. Ultimately the only answer rests in the individual philosophy and conscience of each practitioner. However, some guidelines can be formulated:

1. A placebo should not be given merely as convenience or as a substitute for meaningful doctor–patient communication, in the absence of a carefully established diagnosis, or if it is associated with false information or optimism.
2. On the other hand, placebo interventions may be highly ethical whenever they enhance the doctor–patient relationship or wean the patient away from physical dependence on dangerous drugs. They also are ethical to provide relief to a terminally ill person, by interpolating placebo with active analgesics.

3. Moreover, placebos may play highly useful roles when they are made a part of a careful clinical plan moving the patient actively toward return to a healthy state. This principle can be applied in pain control programs, where a placebo intervention structured into a rehabilitation program may enhance the effort of the pain team to train chronic sufferers to cope with their physical and emotional problems.

REFERENCES

Basbaum, A., and Fields, H. 1978. Endogenous pain control mechanisms: Review and hypothesis. *Ann. Neurol.* 4:1445–1461.

Beecher, H.K. 1961. Surgery as placebo. *JAMA* 176:88–93.

Benson, H., and McCallie, D.P. 1979. Angina pectoris and the placebo effect. *N. Engl. J. Med.* 300:1424–1429.

Chapman, S.L. and Brena, S.F. 1982. Learned helplessness and responses to nerve blocks in chronic low back pain patients. *Pain,* in press.

Diamond, E., and Little, C. 1958. Evaluation of internal mammary artery ligation and sham procedure in angina pectoris. *Circulation* 18:712–713.

Evans, F.J. 1974. The placebo response in pain reduction. *Adv. Neurol.* 4:289–296.

Hartman, K., and Gobel, F. 1976. Effects of placebo on exercise response and nitroglycerine consumption. *Minn. Med.* 59:839–843.

Hillis, B. 1952. The assessment of cough suppressing drugs. *Lancet* 1:1230–1235.

Kadlec, J. 1977. Placebo: A place in medical therapy? *J. Ky. Med. Assoc.* 75:538–540.

Levine, J., Gordon, N., and Fields, H. 1978. The mechanism of placebo analgesia. *Lancet* 2:654–657.

Lyerly, S., Ross, S., Krugman, A., and Clyde J. 1964. The role of placebo instructions. *J. Abnormal Social Psychol.* 69:321–326.

Mintz, I. 1977. A note on the addictive personality: Addiction of placebos. *Am. J. Psychiatr.* 134:327–336.

Moertel, C., Taylor, W., Roth, A., and Tyce, F. 1976. Who responds to sugar pills? *Mayo Clin. Proc.* 57:96–100.

Park, L., and Covi, L. 1965. Nonblind placebo trial. *Arch. Gen. Psychiatr.* 12:336–345.

Pepper, P. 1945. A note on the placebo. *Am. J. Pharmacol.* 117:409–412.

Shapiro, A.P., and Grollman, A. 1953. Critical evaluation of hypotensive action of hydrollazine, hexamethonium, tetraethylammonium, and dibenzyline salts in human and experimental hypertension. *Circulation* 8:188–197.

Sturdebant, R., and Isenberg, J. 1977. Antacid and placebo produced similar pain relief in duodenal ulcer patients. *Gastroenterology* 72:1–5.

Wolf, S., and Pinsky, R.H. 1954. Effects of placebo administration and occurrence of toxic reactions. *JAMA* 155:339–341.

Yonemoto R., Byron, R., and Riihimaki, D. 1975. A double blind prospective study in evaluating narcotics for relief of patients with chronic pain. In *Pain: Research and Treatment,* B.L. Crue (Ed.) New York: Academic Press, pp. 323–325.

20

The Role of the Physical Therapist

BONNIE M. BLOSSOM

Physical therapists need to adapt their treatment methods to the special needs of chronic pain patients. Thus encouraging greater physical function while discouraging pain behaviors becomes an important role for the physical therapist in a behavior modification program. Methods of patient evaluation and treatment are described and ways of recruiting and maintaining staff are discussed.

PHYSICAL THERAPY AND BEHAVIOR MODIFICATION

Considerable success has been experienced by physical therapists in the management of acute and localized pain but the management of chronic pain continues to be a challenge. One discovery made through the years is that individuals with chronic pain do not respond to the conventional treatment modalities and approaches that serve so well in the reduction of acute pain. It therefore has been necessary for the physical therapy practitioner to examine carefully the dynamics of chronic pain by seeking information from other medical specialty groups, such as psychology, and incorporating this information into physical therapy treatment approaches.

Today the approach taken by physical therapists in managing chronic pain is opposite the usual practice of the profession. Many programs follow a behavior modification model, which necessitates the therapist's assuming a fairly rigid and structured attitude and stepping a greater distance away from the patient than is usual and customary. Expression of sympathy and concern, while instrumental in promoting positive outcomes for most clients, can be counterproductive with chronic pain if it serves to reinforce pain behavior. Several physical therapy programs have been successful with behavior modification as the primary base of care in chronic pain management.

NEED AND PHILOSOPHY

It is of critical importance for the physical therapist to seek an understanding of the physician's philosophy of management for the patient with chronic pain and to feel comfortable with that philosophy. The physical therapist then must understand all components of management including methods of referral and the roles of other disciplines and their relationships in carrying out evaluation, treatment, and follow-up. The therapist then is in a position to develop objectives for service that are consistent with the philosophy and objectives of all other disciplines. At Emory University the objective for physical therapy services is to incorporate physical therapy into a behavior modification program designed to increase the patient's functioning. This program is described in Chapter 14.

PROGRAM INDICATORS

Certain program indicators emerge from operant conditioning and from information known about the behavior of chronic pain patients. For example, chronic pain patients tend to focus continuously on their pain. The program, therefore, should direct attention away from the pain, focusing instead on increasing repetitions of exercises, increasing range of motion of specific joint areas, improving tolerance for a particular position or posture, and generally increasing the patient's activity level. Chronic pain patients also are known for their passive role in life, depending upon family members and significant others to think and do for them. Thus the program is conceived so that the patient holds a major responsibility for its implementation. Because many chronic pain patients exercise excessive amounts of inappropriate verbalization of pain, a third program indicator is to ignore and discourage excessive pain behavior.

A fourth indicator arises from the postures that chronic pain patients often assume. If an individual hunches over for prolonged periods of time, sits a lot because it hurts to walk, limps when walking to protect a painful leg, or assumes one or more of a number of bad postural habits, musculoskeletal problems will follow. Therefore, any program design for changing pain behavior should include components to eliminate braces and external support devices when appropriate, strengthen the areas of weakness, increase the areas of limited range of motion, and incorporate these changes into improved static and dynamic postures. Passive means of physical therapy, such as the use of heat and cold, are avoided because they encourage passive dependency and provide only temporary relief. Emphasis is placed instead upon positioning programs for stretching areas of tightness and upon dynamic self-initiated exercises for strengthening muscles, increasing endurance, and promoting good posture.

Because chronic pain patients often focus on themselves, it may be desirable for physical therapy to share space with a general rehabilitation program. By exercising beside an individual with both legs amputated or beside a paralyzed victim of a trampoline accident, pain patients often can put their pain into a better perspective.

EVALUATION

Performing an evaluation is the first step following physician referral. The data base includes a brief social history and a summary of surgical procedures, medical treatment history, past evaluative procedures, other medical problems, and medications. The physical evaluation is extensive and consists of a complete assessment of the strength and range of motion of all extremities, the trunk, and the spine. Spasms and trigger points, responses to deep tendon reflexes, and passive and active straight leg raising are noted. The sensory evaluation includes responses to temperature, to light touch, and to deep pressure. The patient's description of the pain is documented, as well as pain location and observed pain behavior. A functional examination reveals the patient's endurance, activity level, gait, posture, and body mechanics, and the nature and amount of activity of daily living. The activities with which the pain interferes also are noted. Blood pressure, pulse, and respirations are taken at the beginning and end of the evaluation.

TREATMENT

From this evaluation a problem list is generated and goals are established for increasing the activity level, decreasing pain behavior, providing patient education, and improving other specific problems unique to the patient. After discussion of the treatment plan, the patient receives instruction in the type, repetition, and progression of exercises. He/she is given a written home or ward program and is scheduled for daily or weekly monitoring of progress and problems with the therapist, depending on inpatient or outpatient status. During each therapy session, the therapist reviews the patient's monitoring of his or her own daily progress on a graph and advises and encourages. The therapist communicates the results to the appropriate personnel at the pain center on a weekly basis. The form used for this purpose is presented in Table 20-1.

The patient receives exercise documents that include a listing and description of 30 specific exercises. These are listed in categories for the legs, arms, neck, and trunk, and also include exercises using the bicycle, wall pulleys,

Table 20-1
Brief Patient Evaluation Summary

Behavioral Measures (see criteria for ratings)							
Compliance with recommended exercises	very low	1	2	3	4	5	very high
Attention/interest	very low	1	2	3	4	5	very high
Focus on pain	very low	1	2	3	4	5	very high

Joint Mobility
(1 = no joint motion; 2 = ¼ of completed joint ranges; 3 = ½ of completed joint ranged; 4 = ¾ ranged; 5 = normal range)

	Pretreatment					Posttreatment				
Cervical spine	1	2	3	4	5	1	2	3	4	5
Lumbar spine	1	2	3	4	5	1	2	3	4	5
Right upper extremity	1	2	3	4	5	1	2	3	4	5
Left upper extremity	1	2	3	4	5	1	2	3	4	5
Right lower extremity	1	2	3	4	5	1	2	3	4	5
Left lower extremity	1	2	3	4	5	1	2	3	4	5

Muscle Strength
1 = evidence of slight contraction, no joint motion
2 = complete range of motion with gravity eliminated
3 = complete range of motion against gravity
4 = complete range of motion against gravity and some resistance
5 = complete range of motion against gravity with full resistance

	Pretreatment					Posttreatment				
RUE	1	2	3	4	5	1	2	3	4	5
LUE	1	2	3	4	5	1	2	3	4	5
RLE	1	2	3	4	5	1	2	3	4	5
LLE	1	2	3	4	5	1	2	3	4	5
Trunk	1	2	3	4	5	1	2	3	4	5

stairs, and devices used for graded resistive exercises such as the N-K table and the kinetron. After assessing the patient's needs, the therapist specifies the exercises to be performed and indicates the number of repetitions, the frequency, and the duration of each. Goals are set at levels that provide for increasing activity while minimizing risks of failure. As the patient demonstrates success with the recommended program, the therapist adds more exercises and increases repetition and duration of those previously given. At the conclusion of the entire program, the patient may be performing as many as 15 of the exercises or as few as five.

Criteria for "Compliance with Recommended Exercises"

(1) *Very Low* — shows no evidence of doing recommended exercises at home; (2) *Low* — occasionally does recommended exercises at home, but is very inconsistent in adherence to instructions; (3) *Moderate* — usually performs recommended exercises but shows some inconsistency in adherence to instructions; (4) *High* — almost always performs recommended exercises as prescribed; failed to do so only one or two occasions; (5) *Very High* — performs recommended exercises and adheres to instructions 100 percent of the time.

Criteria for "Attention/Interest"

(1) *Very Low* — poor eye contact, no spontaneous questions or comments, provides treatment team with little or no information when requested, shows little evidence of integrating or applying information provided to him; (2) *Low* — few spontaneous questions or comments, when requested, usually provides information or carries out tasks, but with little involvement or enthusiasm, applies only some information provided; (3) *Moderate* — occasionally asks questions or makes comments, provides information or carries out tasks with some involvement or enthusiasm, usually applies information provided; (4) *High* — sometimes asks questions or makes comments, provides information or carries out tasks with involvement and some enthusiasm, complies with treatment suggestions and applies most of information provided; (5) *Very High* — seeks information from many sources, often asks questions and makes comments, not only integrates and applies information provided, but also modifies and extends, carries out tasks with involvement and enthusiasm and shows high level of self-initiative.

Criteria for "Focus on pain"

(1) *Very High* — frequently discusses pain sensations even when not asked, discusses pain repetitively or in highly dramatized terms, nonverbal behavior calls attention to pain, focuses on the things he cannot do because of pain; (2) *High* — sometimes discusses pain sensations when not asked, calls attention frequently to pain through verbal and/or nonverbal behavior, able at times to focus on other aspects of life besides those related to pain; (3) *Moderate* — occasionally focuses attention on pain sensations when not asked, verbal and nonverbal behavior does not usually dramatize the severity of pain, though at times complains about the interference in life brought on by pain, does not do so repetitively; (4) *Low* — very rarely focuses attention on pain sensations when not asked, verbal and nonverbal pain behavior is only seen very intermittently and does not appear dramatized, is able to communicate without making references to pain much of the time; (5) *Very Low* — stoic — shows negligible verbal and nonverbal pain behavior, does not focus on pain sensations when not asked.

STAFFING

The average staff time expended on each patient for each visit is from 40 minutes to one hour. This time includes documentation and communication of results as well as direct patient care. Except for evaluation, review of proper exercise procedures, and medical documentation, the therapist can delegate observation of the patient during exercise and checking the patient's records to a nonprofessional assistant. At Emory a ratio of three professionals to one nonprofessional assistant has worked the best.

RECRUITING AND MAINTAINING STAFF

It is very important that the therapist who works with chronic pain patients understand and accept the unique requirements of working in a highly structured program based on operant conditioning. This type of program provides little or no "hands on" management of the patient. Once the patient is assessed and the program is established, treatment approaches often become routine and the physical therapist may not be stimulated to draw upon the technical knowledge he/she has acquired through extensive professional training. As a result it is usually beneficial for therapists assigned to the pain team to work with patients with other problems besides pain, with whom they can be less stiff and businesslike.

Continuing professional education also helps maintain staff by providing greater job satisfaction and by helping therapists stay in tune with advancing knowledge in many areas of physical therapy. Staff morale also improves when therapists can make use of nonprofessional aides to carry on tasks that are routine and do not require professional judgment.

The opportunity to share ideas about program improvement and to function as an integral part of a cohesive staff also is vital. Each discipline must work together toward common goals, and progress in reaching these goals must be demonstrated through careful and continual evaluation.

BIBLIOGRAPHY

Fordyce, W.E. 1976. *Behavioral Methods for Chronic Pain and Illness*. St. Louis: C.V. Mosby.

Fordyce, W.E., Fowler, R.S., Lehman, J.F., and DeLateur, B.J. 73. Operant conditioning in the treatment of chronic pain. *Arch. Phys. Med. Rehab.* 54:399–408.

Meilman, P.W. 1979. Psychological aspects of chronic pain. *J. Orthopaed. Sports Phys. Therap.* 1:76–82.

Roesch, R., and Ulrich, D.E. 1980. Physical therapy management in the treatment of chronic pain. *Phys. Therap.* 60:53–57.

21

The Role of the Occupational Therapist

BETTE A. GROAT

Occupational therapy plays a significant role in the team treatment of the chronic pain patient. It is instrumental in teaching interpersonal and self-management skills required to cope adequately with the demands of living. By the concentrated emphasis on the chronic pain patients' strengths and abilities instead of on their impairment, the occupational therapist helps them find ways to gain the satisfaction of being involved and productive.

Occupational therapy's central focus is the self-directed, productive behavior of human beings, and thus it bases its rationale on developmental processes fundamental to growth and creativity (Willard & Spackman, 1971). Coupled with this foundation is the philosophy that activities form an integral part of everyday life and are the tools through which human beings learn and develop. As individuals engage in an activity, they explore their interests, needs, capabilities, and limitations, develop skills, and learn a range of interpersonal and social attitudes and behaviors. Success in activities provides them with immediate and concrete evidence of their ability to be productive. Moreover, by participation in appropriate activities an individual is given an elementary source of satisfaction necessary for a healthy self-image (American Occupational Therapy Association, 1972). The success of this combination was most adequately described by Diasio (1968): "... one of the distinguishing features of occupational therapy is its conscious emphasis and insistence that in addition to man's need for meaningful engagement with his environment, there are therapeutic properties inherent in the environment which may be structured for treatment purposes" (page 400).

Many chronic pain patients have allowed their lives to become so much determined by their pain syndrome that they have lost a sense of what they can do. Furthermore, major imbalances of work, rest, and play often have developed. The occupational therapist can structure activities and discussions to help the patient realize his/her potential and achieve the balance associated with healthy living.

This chapter presents a comprehensive occupational therapy program that can be used to meet these goals with the chronic pain patient. Participation of the therapist in the program can be divided into five parts: (1) individual patient assessment and evaluation; (2) therapeutic group activities; (3) appropriate treatment for decreased functional capacities as identified in the evaluation; (4) family education; and (5) involvement as a team member in achieving a comprehensive program for the chronic pain patient.

OCCUPATIONAL THERAPY EVALUATION

Each patient seen in the pain control center is referred to occupational therapy. Upon referral the occupational therapist interviews the patient individually in order to begin to develop therapeutic trust and rapport and to gain a broad overview of the following problem areas.

Living Situation

This evaluation of both the family structure and physical structure within the home environment allows identification of both the patient's emotional support systems and possible architectural barriers.

Education/Work Experience

The therapist evaluates possible monetary reinforcement for pain behavior, job skills, experience, and abilities, and the patient's percepton of his/her vocational and educational needs and problems.

Functional Status

The patients are evaluated for any physical incapacities that hinder their functional ability in the areas of self-care, homemaking, and mobility. Most important, it is determined whether patients currently are performing these functions.

Activity Configuration

A typical day's activities are outlined and the amount of past and present participation in each listed activity is determined.

Coping Skills

The patients' present modes for handling stress are explored to determine if stressful events have become debilitating and whether a positive self-concept has been maintained. In addition the patients' basic ability to process information effectively is assessed.

Appearance/Self-Expression/Attitude

A gross initial assessment is made of whether the patient assumes responsibility for his/her action and feelings; whether there is recognition of his/her strengths, weaknesses, and limitations; how he/she feels others view him/her; and whether personal hygiene has been maintained.

TREATMENT GOALS

Upon completion of the evaluation, a problem list is compiled for each patient. This list suggests work toward one or more of the following general treatment objectives: (1) to increase awareness of personal values; (2) to develop effective problem-solving behavior; (3) to increase self-esteem; (4) to develop balance in work/play/rest relationships; (5) to learn and apply techniques of stress management and relaxation; (6) to increase assertiveness; (7) to improve life skills in areas of work, self-maintenance, socialization, and use of free time; (8) to alleviate depression; (9) to improve upper extremity function (desensitization, strength, range of motion, function); and (10) to increase independence in specific activities of daily living (bathing, dressing, homemaking, etc.).

Occupational therapy treatment is conducted individually and in groups. The last two treatment objectives are generally scheduled individually; the others are addressed in the Life Skills Program conducted in groups.

LIFE SKILLS PROGRAM

The Life Skills Program consists of experiential learning tasks in a group setting based on a learning competency model (Thomas and Bujema, 1977). This model comprises three elements; competency, initiative, and self-esteem. Thomas and Bujema postulate that these elements are dependent on and interrelate with each other (Fig. 21-1).

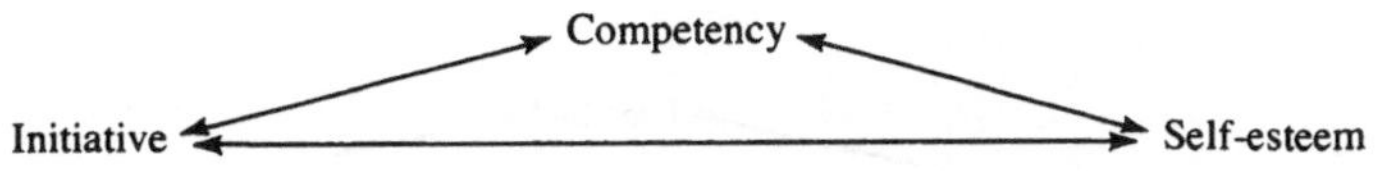

FIG. 21-1. Learning competency model.

Through competent behavior an individual gains recognition, thus building self-esteem. Self-esteem predisposes the individual to initiate further behavior and to learn from the environment, which adds to his/her repertoire of skills. By this process acceptable adaptive behavior is acquired.

Discussion among participants is an important part of these groups; however, no attempt is made to delve into past histories or unresolved hidden conflicts. Pain behavior is discouraged while discussion of positive methods of coping is reinforced. Patients are expected to participate actively and discuss how the underlying principles can be incorporated into their individual life-styles.

Inpatients and outpatients on the intensive two-week program attend these groups Monday through Friday on a daily basis. All other outpatients attend once a week for six weeks. There is one occupational therapist per group of 8 to 12 patients and each session is one hour in duration. Basic subjects discussed in the therapeutic groups are coping with stress, balancing daily activities, goal setting/decision making, interpersonal relationships, and self-management. Goal setting/decision making is generally discussed in two sessions, while the other topics each involves one group session.

Coping with Stress

It is emphasized that stressors are changes that can be big or small and desired or not desired; they are not necessarily bad or good. Studies have shown that when individuals experience a large number of changes in a short period of time, they proportionally raise the risk of illness and/or accidents (see Chapter 15). Chronic pain patients must develop the ability to identify not only what their daily stressors are, but also what their reactions are to these stressors. Once different types of stressors and reactions have been identified, the occupational therapist actively elicits discussion of each patient's own coping mechanisms and their effectiveness for long-term usage. The therapist then instructs the group in possible adaptive responses to stress (i.e., constructive physical activity, relaxation techniques, etc.).

Balancing Activities

Chronic pain patients frequently display an imbalance in their activities between work, rest, and play, and often are trapped in a decreased activity cycle (Fig. 21-2).

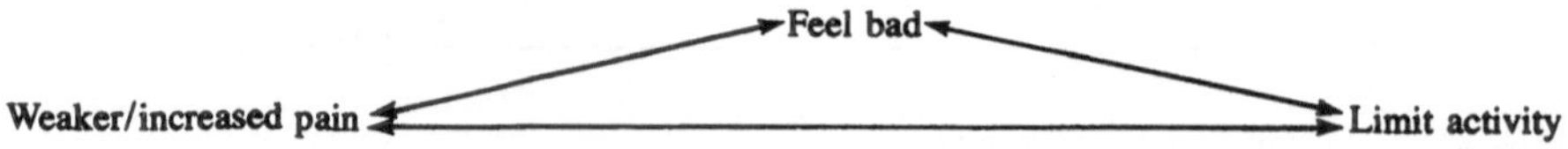

FIG. 21-2. Decreased activity cycle.

During this group patients outline their typical day's activities prior to treatment. They then grade each activity as to the type (work, rest, or play) how well they performed it, the level of satisfaction it gave them, and how much time they devoted to it. The occupational therapist encourages each group member to determine the type of activities missing in his/her own life. Individuals then must identify changes they want to make, and develop and write the action steps necessary to achieve these changes. The goal is to teach the patient that he/she can be a positive change agent in modifying everyday activities so as to achieve a balanced schedule to decrease stress and to increase health and happiness.

Goal Setting/Decision Making

Since their world centers around pain and they feel little, if any, control over it, many chronic pain patients feel helpless and thus unmotivated to seek change. To break this vicious cycle, the occupational therapist encourages the patient to write down achievable goals and priorities, and to develop specific steps for this achievement. The mere presence of such goals reduces helplessness and hopelessness.

Another method by which chronic pain patients can gain additional control in their lives is through strengthening of their decision-making skills. One task that can be employed is to ask each group member (including the therapist) to write down one decision he/she is facing and is willing to share with the group. The whole group then brainstorms on alternative answers, and each alternative is examined to determine its pros and cons. Although this process represents nothing more than simple problem solving, it is new and useful to most chronic pain patients.

Interpersonal Relationships

For effective interaction with their environment, individuals must establish communication modes that will meet their needs. Many chronic pain patients assume a passive or aggressive role in communication. In addition much of their communication is in the language of pain, which sometimes is used as an indirect means to express needs for help or attention or to express anger and resentment. In the groups the patients are taught the open communication of assertiveness through which needs and feelings can be expressed while still considering the needs and feelings of others. The chronic pain patients are instructed that assertiveness promotes self-respect and self-esteem.

Self-Management

This group focuses on ways of increasing self-awareness and self-esteem. It explores the factors that can prolong illness and identifies alternative wellness-oriented behavior modes through which chronic pain patients can meet their needs. One factor explored in this group is the feeling of uselessness common in chronic pain patients. Patients are encouraged to list areas in which they are very capable, worthy, and successful. For example, they may express disappointment in not being able to maintain a full-time job, but they may be carrying out tasks at home that help the total family.

Family Education

Families are included in the Life Skills groups whenever possible, and methods by which they cope with the pressures of the patient's illnes are discussed. Because the family's responses to the patient at home are critical for maintaining changes, families are encouraged to reinforce the patient to put into action the principles discussed in the groups.

PERSPECTIVES ON THE LIFE SKILLS PROGRAM

The Life Skills groups have provided a positive experience for patients in that they focus on positive methods of coping and provide needed socialization for the patients. To maintain the staff interest and enthusiasm necessary to maintain effectiveness, it has been necessasry to rotate group leaders every three to six months to prevent "burnout." Rotating leaders and scheduling more groups to maintain small numbers in each group have helped to avoid projecting a feeling of mass production despite a large patient load.

FUNCTIONAL CAPACITIES TREATMENT

If the initial evaluation revealed physical deficits that limit function, a suitable individual occupational therapy program may be designed using graded activities and exercise to improve any problems identified. This program may focus on such daily activities as self-care, including feeding, dressing, and hygiene; homemaking, including cooking, cleaning, management, home maintenance, and yard work; and recreational and vocational activities. If special equipment (such as splints or self-care devices) is required that makes it easier or safer to do things, it is provided and the occupational therapist trains the patient in its use and care.

The majority of chronic pain patients receive instruction in the principles of work simplification, joint protection, and body mechanics. This instruction is important, as patients otherwise might limit or avoid activities in fear of hurting themselves further. Areas of focus might include correct working heights for tasks requiring standing or sitting, how to allow gravity to work for one, how to avoid unduly stressing joints, and how to plan better activities for energy conservation.

Occupational therapist's impressions of ______________________

Does not attend groups	0	1	2	3	4	Attends groups regularly
Seems disinterested	0	1	2	3	4	Actively participates
Negative attitude	0	1	2	3	4	Positive attitude
Does not understand concepts	0	1	2	3	4	Understands concepts
Lacks insight	0	1	2	3	4	Insightful

(See occupational therapist's discharge note for complete data.)

FIG. 21-3. Evaluation of patient progress in Life Skills.

TEAMWORK

Teamwork is the vehicle through which a comprehensive and consistent program is maintained for the patients. It becomes especially critical in the management of difficult, distrustful, or manipulative patients. Like all members of the treatment team, occupational therapists maintain teamwork through daily communications about problems, structured weekly staff meetings, and regular inservice education about chronic pain. Having all services in close physical proximity helps maintain this needed close communication. Fig. 21-3 presents a simple form placed in the patient's chart to communicate information about the progress of patients in the Life Skills group.

REFERENCES

American Occupational Therapy Association 1972. Special Task Force. *Am. J. Occupat. Therap.* 22:400.

Diasio, K. 1968. Psychiatric occupational therapy: Search for a conceptual framework in light of psycho-analytic ego psychology and learning theory. *Am. J. Occupat. Therap.* 26:204–205.

Thomas, L.J., and Bajema, S.L. 1974. Unpublished. Occupational Therapy Life Skills Development Program proposed at Dwight David Eisenhower Army Medical Center, Fort Gordon, Ga.

Willard, H.S., and Spackman, C.S. 1971. *Occupational Therapy*. Philadelphia: J.B. Lippincott.

22

Legal Aspects of Pain and Disability

HOWARD I. GROSSMAN

Differences in the administration of Workers' Compensation and Social Security payments are presented. In many ways the rules of evidence in Social Security cases permit distortions and unjustified disability grants. Because of the potential for immense personal, social, and economic loss in disability grants, physicians must be aware of the issues and be careful in their assessments and reports.

Editors' note: Throughout this book the impact of pending disability claims or actual disability benefits has been discussed. Over half of the chronic sufferers interviewed at many pain control facilities in the United States are receiving disability compensation or have applied for them. Professionals in general practice and even on the staff of pain control facilities rarely are aware that their observations, assessments, and recommendations sooner or later will be reviewed, dissected, and interpreted not according to their medical meaning but according to the goals set by the adversaries in a court of law. Because of the lack of agreement about assessment of pain, impairment, and disability, the outcome of the legal process in disability cases is not so much related to actual medical findings but to the intepretation (or distortion) of such findings by opposing attorneys.

It is imperative that professionals at pain control facilities who accept the responsibility to evaluate and treat chronic sufferers also accept the responsibility to provide them with comprehensive assessments of impairment and disability. This assessment will increase the likelihood of a fair decision in court. Basic principles of impairment and disability evaluations are presented in Chapter 10. This chapter provides the general practitioner an insight into the legal issues relating to chronic pain, and the role of physicians' reports in determining the outcome of disability cases.

WORKERS' COMPENSATION AND SOCIAL SECURITY

There are three principal forms of compensation for accidental injury and illness in the United States: Workers' Compensation, dependent largely on state laws as well as on two federal statutes; disability benefits under the federal Social Security Act; and private disability insurance policies.

These benefit systems had their beginnings in different circumstances. Workers' Compensation laws were passed because of dissatisfaction with employee rights in cases of work-related injury, illness, or death. The employer had defenses based on the concept that the employee had to prove that the employer was "at fault" for the injury, which made it difficult or impossible for the employee to collect. In the late 19th and early 20th centuries, a new idea developed that work-related injuries and illnesses were a "social cost" of industrialization, and that liability should be imposed on the employer "without fault." It was assumed that the employer, in turn, passed along these costs to the public in the form of higher prices. Financing of Workers' Compensation is accomplished most frequently by the use of private insurance carriers, although state funds are sometimes used, and in some instances employers can prove their capacity for "self-insurance."

Unlike Workers' Compensation laws, disability benefits under the Social Security Act need not be based upon a work-related impairment. In order to finance this system, Social Security taxes are collected from employees, employers, and self-employed persons working in jobs and businesses covered by the Act. Some of these taxes then are paid into the Federal Disability Insurance Trust Fund. To qualify for Disability Insurance benefits, a worker must have worked a certain minimum period of time.

Though Workers' Compensation benefits vary from state to state according to their individual laws, federal benefits are uniform in all states; however, they do vary widely from individual to individual depending upon age at disability and past earnings. The same person can receive both kinds of benefits at the same time, but the Social Security Act provides that disability benefits will be reduced whenever the combination of state and federal benefits exceeds 80 percent of the worker's average earnings or the family's total Social Security benefits.

Responsibility for application for benefits under both systems lies with the injured or sick individual. Under most Workers' Compensation laws, the worker must notify his/her employer of the injury within a specified time, usually 30 days. If the worker does not receive benefits, he/she must file a claim with the State Board of Workers' Compensation, usually within one year from the date of the accident. The worker is entitled under most state laws to a hearing before an administrative law judge.

Under the Social Security Act, the worker must file an application for Disability Insurance benefits at a local Social Security district office. If the claim is denied, there are successive levels of appeal to an administrative law judge and ultimately to the federal courts.

The definition of disability and the waiting time for payment vary under state and federal laws. State laws provide for temporary total disability, permanent total disability, and permanent partial disability. As with benefits administered by the Veterans Administration, disability is often given a percentage rating and benefits are paid accordingly. The worker generally is entitled to benefits after a short period of time, usually one week. Under the Social Security Act, however, disability is total and is defined as inability to work because of a medical impairment. To receive disability the person must be evaluated as unable to work for a period of time that has lasted or can be expected to last for one year. In addition the worker must wait five months after being disabled before getting benefits.

As a result of these differences, Workers' Compensation cases more typically involve short-term impairments such as acute illnesses or accidents susceptible to remedial treatment, whereas Social Security cases include more chronic impairments. In recent years there has been an increase in Workers' Compensation awards for stress on the job. The Supreme Court of Michigan recently granted lifetime Workers Compensation to a parts inspector on a General Motors production line, because he was a "perfectionist" who suffered stress when assembly line workers insisted on installing a part he had labeled defective.

Awarding Workers' Compensation benefits on the basis of mental impairments would lead to an increase in costs. It would also lend credence to the arguments of critics who contend that it is impracticable to separate occupational from nonoccupational disability. Of greater significance, it would extend the problem of proof of disability, which already exists in federal Social Security cases, to Workers' Compensation cases.

ASSESSING PROOF OF DISABILITY

The Social Security Administration evaluates cases according to both a claimant's statement about his/her pain and inability to function and according to "objective medical evidence" such as diagnoses, laboratory test results, and records of treatment. However, they suspend some rules of evidence used in private injury cases and as a result allow some individuals to receive unjustified disability benefits.

Rules of evidence in ordinary private injury cases prevent the introduction of evidence found in doctor's reports that are based on the claimant's statements. This hearsay rule requires that a witness base any statements on his/her own knowledge rather than on a claimant's statements. Witnesses thus can be cross-examined to ensure that judgments are accurate and truthful and based on their own knowledge.

In private injury cases, an exception is made to the hearsay rule in the case of a patient who sees a doctor solely for treatment, because it is assumed that the patient would have every reason to tell the truth; however, the doctor's opinion based on a litigant's statements is barred if this opinion was sought for testimony in a lawsuit. As stated by a Texas court, "to permit the expert's opinion based upon such statements . . . to go before the jury, would open the door for the grossest fraud . . .''*

The rules for Social Security cases not only allow such testimony, but encourage it by providing for ''consultative examinations'' with a doctor designated by a state agency specifically to see if the worker is entitled to monetary payments. In these cases the doctor is not involved in treatment and thus the patient has no reason to do anything else but report symptoms so as to maximize the chances for a favorable outcome in litigation. The Social Security regulations do not distinguish between the validity of reports from treating or consultative physicians; if anything, a greater weight is attached to the consultative reports. In addition no distinction is made between reports filed from treating physicians before or after a disability claim is filed.

The regulations do provide that the statement of a doctor that an individual is or is not disabled is not ''determinative'' of the issue of disability, but is to be given weight to the extent that it is supported by clinical evidence. Although useful this regulation does not make the fine distinctions needed in difficult problems of credibility.

Difficulties are illustrated by the common case of a minor or nonexistent physical impairment exacerbated by mental illness. The psychiatrist's report documents the mental illness, but may be based on the claimant's appearance, demeanor, and thought processes as manifested by what he/she says. A psychiatrist who believes those words as representing objective facts may make a finding of ''psychophysiological reaction,'' which is accepted at the hearing as scientific evidence. What has happened is that the claimant's statements have been bolstered by an expert based on the expert's belief that what the claimant says is true. It is important for the psychiatrist to realize that Social Security regulations identify and describe mental disorders as organic brain syndromes, functional mental disorders (psychotic, psychophysiologic, psychoneurotic, and personality disorders), and mental deficiency. Making such a diagnosis can easily result in the granting of disability benefits. Typically cases involving psychiatric diagnosis with suspicion of functional complaints and absence of objective findings become bogged down in confusion, appeals, and expensive litigation.

Another issue not addressed is the effect of the doctor's statements on the patient. A doctor who tells a patient he or she is too sick to work is usually believed, and the patient might *become* too sick to work as a result.

The problem of distorted evidence in Social Security cases is compounded by the absence of an adversary proceeding at the hearing level. Almost half the claimants appear with competent attorneys knowledgeable about the laws of evidence or lack of any law in Social Security cases; however, no attorney will be

*Texas Employer's Inc. Assoc. v. Wallace, 70 SW 2d 833 (Tex. Civ. App., 1934)

assigned to defend the fund of taxpayer's money, even though each case has an actuarial value of about $100,000. The Administrative Law Judge is supposed to defend the fund against unjust attacks but, on the other hand, is also supposed to help the claimant develop a case in order to get money from the fund. How can the judge do both? An ALJ who tries vigorous cross-examination of a claimant—which should be the job of opposing counsel—is accused of bias on judicial review and is reversed.

A bill sponsored by Administrative Law Judges that attempted to correct some of these deficiencies was opposed by the Social Security Administration and was not reflected in the Social Security Disability Amendments of 1980. This bill would have provided for "lesser probative weight" for physicians' opinions after the filing of disability and for greater weight to be given to psychiatric opinions that distinguish between verbal assertions of the claimant and objective evidence of mental illness. To avoid unjustified disability benefits, professionals must be careful to distinguish in their reports between what the patient said and what objective evidence indicated and to base their judgments about disability on the latter.

Many physicians prefer to "wash their hands" of the disability issue and leave it to the attorneys. They often forget that disability determination might then be made by people less expert than themselves. Moreover, many of them fail to realize the human, social, and economic wastage involved in cases of young people with mild injuries who receive disability and remain idle except to have periodic expensive medical treatments. Any person who accepts disability income without good reason is likely to deteriorate physically and emotionally. Such disability fosters passivity and helplessness, as recipients give up control of their lives and become dependent on a faceless bureaucratic system.

Closing Remarks

STEVEN F. BRENA, AND STANLEY L. CHAPMAN

Throughout this book the phenomenon of pain has been discussed in its complexity from different perspectives. Pertinent research findings have been translated into a language that may be easily understood by the average medical and paramedical professional. Several key points that are crucial to a circular understanding of human pain have been presented and are here briefly summarized with a few closing remarks.

1. Pain is a universal phenomenon that is deeply embedded in the very nature of all living creatures. In its acute, pathogenic form, the painful experience seems to have a meaningful biological value as a warning signal of a homeostatic derangement. In its chronic manifestation, pain seems to have lost any biological dignity, to the point that it may evolve into a destructive, self-sustaining, existential disease.

Far from being "benign," chronic pain heavily taxes the endurance of the individual sufferer. Along the teaching of the Orientals, it could be argued that a prolonged painful experience may still have the meaning of a useful "signal," warning that something is "wrong" and "imbalanced" in our "cosmic" homeostasis, not only at the biological level, but at higher existential levels also. Within the Judeo-Christian tradition, chronic pain may be viewed as having a redeeming dignity, as a challenge to the sufferer to rise above unpleasant sensory perceptions and seek compensation in higher intellectual and spiritual values. Clinically, the problem is contained when the sufferer's competent coping is preserved; however, when the individual's coping skills break down, the suffering increases and cries for help go out to the health professionals and to the "good neighbor." Almost paradoxically many well-motivated professional and social responses to the anguished cries of the human sufferer seem to strengthen the painful experience by creating or exacerbating maladaptive illness behaviors (learned pain).

2. The central nervous system is a powerful living computer capable of storing information received from the outside, integrating it, and providing adaptive responses. Well-integrated behaviors are a function of the "black box," in terms of thoughts, feelings, and values. Inhibitory neurochemical circuit breakers seem to play significant roles in modulating and processing sensory

overloads. At present the painful perception, mostly in its pathogenic form, seems to be at least partially influenced by these inhibitory mechanisms.

Loss of antinociceptive inhibition may be a causative factor of the painful experience, at least at its onset. Breakdown factors include biological dysfunctions, emotional maladjustments, and ecological stressors; they may be both preexisting—possibly even at the genetic level—and generated by the sensory overload itself. The stabilizing role of the black box has to be better understood. At present, clinical experience from the pain control centers of the United States points out that the tampering with the central nervous system by overprescription of medication is a major stressor leading to breakdown.

3. The musculoskeletal system has evolved to provide the animal with driving mechanisms for survival and reproduction. Vascular and visceral systems evolved mainly for a single purpose: to nourish the muscles and keep them functional. In humans the muscular system also provides emotional expressions by translating feelings into movements. Muscular function is therefore closely associated with vascular–visceral and psychological stability, in a two-way relationship.

Musculoskeletal activation into a "fight or flight reaction" is the main survival tool in mammals; observation of animal life shows that this primordial survival mechanism has the capability to function even in the presence of severe nociceptive insults, to be followed by a period of inactivity for healing of the injuries only after the survival challenge is over. Prolonged inactivity, biologically unjustified in the presence of static, tonic nociception or in the absence of nociceptive stimulation, leads to severe muscular, visceral, and emotional malfunctions, which are at the very source of chronic pain. Well-documented results from the major pain control centers show beyond reasonable doubts that restoration of musculoskeletal activity to normality through behavioral rehabilitation leads to consistent physical and emotional improvements of chronic sufferers. On the other hand, medical intervention supporting biologically useless inactivity contributes heavily to the morbidity of chronic pain.

4. Traditional medical diagnostic investigation mainly directed toward the detection of biological abnormality is very inadequate in the diagnosis, assessment, and classification of chronic pain states. A multidimensional approach aimed at the investigation of biological, psychological, and social variables is imperative to reach meaningful levels of probability. The black box model is a useful operational definition of chronic pain, upon which most assessment strategies are based. At present there is no diagnostic method for chronic pain assessment that has gained nationwide acceptance. The Emory Pain Estimate Model has been operative since 1975, has been repeatedly tested both at Emory and at other pain control centers, and has been found valid and reliable, but is not (yet) a standard procedure for the diagnosis of chronic pain.

Major roadblocks on the way to reaching an acceptable standard methodology for chronic pain assessment include incomplete knowledge of the functioning of the nociceptive systems; fragmentary and controversial findings relating to biological malfunctions of the musculoskeletal system and the related connective system; resistance within the medical profession to recognize the perceptual and emotional dimensions of pain and an even greater resistance to accept, integrate, and apply research findings from behavioral science; an enormous semantic confusion, by which many professionals are driven to label the same clinical observation with different names, while rarely agreeing on the real meaning of many of them; and mammoth confusion in reaching reliability and validity in the evaluation of impairment and disability of pain-disabled patients, which feeds the unacceptable cost of chronic pain on the legal and social levels.

5. No single treatment modality capable of long-term control of chronic pain is presently available. The key factor in restoring chronic pain patients to a lasting state of health probably is the "reprogramming of the black box" through multimodal intervention upon the nervous system and the musculoskeletal system. While such intervention is targeted at the pain location, its long-term goal is the training of the whole individual in new adaptive skills effectively to cope with whatever biological, emotional, and social abnormality has been detected. Treatment outcome reports from reputable pain control centers do show much promise in these treatment strategies.

Obstacles to this approach include the busy nature of general practice, rightly concerned with saving lives by aggressive intervention in cases of acute biological derangements; the inadequate or nonexistent training of general practitioners in behavior and rehabilitation medicine and their reluctance to learn even some basic principles; the medical overreliance on external intervention (drugs and techniques) for management of complex health problems; the societal expectation that such complex health problems may be "fixed" through technical and chemical manipulation; and the present structure of the practice of medicine itself, with the inevitable tunnel-vision approach to health problems within strict speciality boundaries.

6. The question of evaluating the competency of mushrooming pain control facilities in the United States is often raised. At present there are no nationwide guidelines for the recognition and certification of pain control facilities.* The recommendations of an *ad hoc* committee of the American Pain Society to study ways to provide such certification have been presented to the board of directors.

*In its 1983 "Standards Manual for Facilities Serving People with Disabilities," C.A.R.F. (*Commission on Accreditation of Rehabilitation Facilities*) will provide a special section which sets guidelines for certification of Pain Control and Rehabilitation Facilities. These guidelines have been proposed by a special National Advisory Committee, which met in Chicago in July 1982.

Currently the only valid criteria by which to gauge the operation of a pain control facility are to examine its methods for pain evaluation, classification, and monitoring of outcome of treatment. The complexity of pain problems makes it imperative to have proper and efficient monitoring of progress reports from patients, other than verbal changes in pain complaints only. Failure to provide a sound and organized monitoring system may lead to delusive assessments of improvements and may actually harm the chronic sufferer. A competent pain control facility will have a monitoring operation wide open to peer evaluation and information. Monitoring techniques have been discussed throughout this book.

Misconceptions, obstacles, and roadblocks may be removed; actually this refreshing process has started already:

a. The International Association for Study of Pain (IASP) has set up a committee on "taxonomy," with the precise intent of reviewing and redefining old medical terms into new definitions that better reflect present-day knowledge. The same committee has also been charged to provide guidelines for improved assessment of chronic pain states.

b. While not yet professionally recognized, a new breed of health professionals, with special training in behavior and rehabilitation medicine built upon a sound and circular general medical knowledge, is taking over the operation of pain control facilities in the United States and in many other countries; this new practice of medicine aimed at chronic pain problems has been called "algology—the science of pain management." The special *ad hoc* committee of the American Pain Society (APS) for accreditation of pain control facilities has informally recognized the existence and viability of algology, and has made the recommendation to the APS board of directors for its official recognition.

c. The IASP and the APS have generated a tremendous momentum for enhancing education and research on pain. Throughout the world, and especially in the United States, educational courses on pain are offered, to give the practitioner of every medical speciality an opportunity to learn "new coping skills" with which to deal with chronic pain patients.

d. While the management of chronic pain patients, mostly in cases of learned pain, should be the field of algology practice, the general practitioner who has gained proper information and skill can play active roles in the prevention of learned pain and in the effective treatment of some chronic sufferers. Guidelines for such roles in general practice have been discussed throughout this book, especially in Chapters 2, 11, and 12.

In summary chronic pain represents a disease in itself, with characteristics and associated treatments very different from any other set of problems within the field of medicine, including psychiatry. Because the human wastage represented by this disease is massive, it is the challenge of the health professional from every medical and paramedical speciality to recognize it, understand its unique concepts, and help prevent it and treat those who suffer from it so that they can be restored to healthy and productive lives.

Index